BILIARY CHOLANGITIS COOKBOOK

HEALTHY RECIPES TO MANAGE THRIVING LIVER DISEASES FOR QUICK RECOVERY

KAREN EDMONDS

TABLE OF CONTENT

INTRODUCTION..7

CHAPTER 1: UNDERSTANDING BILIARY CHOLANGITIS........................9

Importance of Diet in Managing Biliary Cholangitis 12

CHAPTER 2: OVERVIEW OF THE BILIARY CHOLANGITIS DIET: 15

CHAPTER 2: BREAKFAST DELIGHTS 19

Keto Sausage Egg Cups 19

Blueberry Compote Oatmeal..............24

Dandelion Greens Sauté 29

CHAPTER 3: APPETIZERS FOR OPTIMAL DIGESTION........................35

Avocado and Tomato Bruschetta.......35

Cucumber Rolls with Hummus..........40

Beetroot and Walnut Dip 45

CHAPTER 4: NOURISHING SOUPS AND SALADS 51

Healthy Chicken Noodle Soup.............51

Springtime Salad with Chicken and Berries 56

Roasted Cauliflower & Potato Curry Soup 61

CHAPTER 5: SATISFYING MAIN DISHES 67

Baked Salmon with Dill Sauce 67

Turkey and Vegetable Stir-Fry 72

Lentil and Sweet Potato Shepherd's Pie 78

CHAPTER 6: SIDE DISHES AND SNACKS 85

Crispy Baked Zucchini Fries 90

Almond and Date Energy Balls 96

CHAPTER 7: DESSERT OPTIONS ...101

Berry Chia Seed Pudding 101

Dark Chocolate Avocado Mousse 106

Baked Apples with Cinnamon and Walnuts 111

CHAPTER 8 117

Liver Lovin' Smoothie 117

Green Beauty Cilantro Shake...........121

Healthy "Shamrock" Shake 126

4-3-2-1 Green Smoothie...................131

Bok Choy Green Smoothie...............135

Golden Turmeric Latte Smoothie 140

Dandelion Beetroot juice..................145

Blast of broccoli smoothie 149

....149

Lemon-Lime Coconut Smoothie.......153

Banana Chocolate Smoothie 158

Green machine smoothie...................163

Green Detox Smoothie......................167

CHAPTER 9 173

Adapting recipes for special dietary needs 173

CHAPTER 10: 7 DAY MEAL PLAN..177

CHAPTER 11: CONCLUSION 179

Bonus 181

INTRODUCTION

Welcome to the Biliary Cholangitis Cookbook, where great dishes meet sensible nutritional choices to help you on your health journey! If you live with biliary cholangitis, you understand how vital it is to nourish your body with foods that promote wellbeing. This cookbook will help you create delicious meals that not only satisfy your taste buds but also support your liver and general health.

Biliary cholangitis, also known as primary biliary cholangitis (PBC), is a chronic liver disease affecting the bile ducts. These tiny tubes transport bile, a fluid generated by the liver, to the small intestine for digestion. Bile duct injury and inflammation can cause a variety of symptoms, including weariness, itching, and digestive difficulties. While there is no treatment for biliary cholangitis, changing your diet can improve your quality of life and delay the course of the condition.

This cookbook is a treasure mine of recipes that have been carefully selected to meet your nutritional demands. Each recipe, from substantial breakfasts to filling main courses and decadent desserts, is created with health in mind. We have added nourishing foods that are mild on the liver and high in critical nutrients to help you feel your best.

However, this cookbook is more than simply recipes; it is a comprehensive resource that will help you understand the significance of nutrition in biliary cholangitis treatment. You will discover helpful hints for meal planning, portion management, and modifying recipes to your specific dietary tastes and needs. So, whether you have just been diagnosed or are a seasoned fighter in the fight against biliary cholangitis, let this cookbook be your culinary partner on the road to improved health and vigour.

CHAPTER 1:
UNDERSTANDING BILIARY CHOLANGITIS

Biliary cholangitis, or primary biliary cholangitis (PBC), is a chronic liver illness that causes inflammation and damage to the liver's tiny bile ducts. The bile ducts transfer bile, a digestive fluid generated by the liver, to the small intestine. Biliary cholangitis occurs when the immune system wrongly assaults and destroys the bile ducts, eventually destroying them. As a result, bile accumulates in the liver, producing further inflammation, scarring (cirrhosis), and decreased liver function.

Symptoms of Biliary Cholangitis:

The symptoms of biliary cholangitis can vary greatly across individuals and may develop gradually. Common symptoms include:

Fatigue: Persistent weariness and a lack of energy are prominent early indicators of biliary cholangitis.

Itching (Pruritus): Itching, especially on the hands and feet, is a typical symptom caused by bile salt accumulation in the circulation.

Jaundice: Yellowing of the skin and eyes can be caused by a build-up of bilirubin, a yellow pigment in the body.

Abdominal Discomfort: Some people may feel discomfort or pain in the upper right side of their abdomen, where the liver resides.

Dry Eyes and Mouth: Less production of tears and saliva might cause dry eyes and mouth.

Complications from Biliary Cholangitis:

If left untreated, biliary cholangitis can lead to significant problems such as:

Cirrhosis: Chronic inflammation and scarring of the liver might eventually result in liver failure.

Osteoporosis*:* Poor absorption of fat-soluble vitamins and decreased bile flow can increase the risk of osteoporosis and fractures.

Malabsorption: Malnutrition can result from bile duct dysfunction that prevents lipids and fat-soluble vitamins from being absorbed.

Portal Hypertension: Liver scarring can raise pressure in the portal vein, leading to problems such as varices (enlarged veins) and ascites.

Individuals with biliary cholangitis must work closely with healthcare providers to control symptoms, decrease disease progression, and avoid complications via lifestyle changes, medicines, and regular monitoring.

Importance of Diet in Managing Biliary Cholangitis

The role of food in controlling biliary cholangitis cannot be emphasised. Biliary cholangitis is a chronic liver illness that necessitates careful dietary choices in order to relieve symptoms, decrease disease progression, and enhance general health and well-being.

Liver Support: The liver regulates bile production and detoxifying activities. A diet high in minerals, antioxidants, and healthy fats can help improve liver function and reduce inflammation, which is essential for controlling biliary cholangitis.

Bile Flow Regulation: Damage to the bile ducts in biliary cholangitis can impair bile flow, causing problems. Certain dietary changes, such as eating foods rich in soluble fibre and healthy fats, can help regulate bile flow and avoid bile accumulation in the liver.

Nutritional Balance: Individuals with biliary cholangitis may suffer from nutritional deficits as a result of poor bile absorption. A well-balanced diet rich in protein, vitamins, minerals, and vital fatty acids is critical for good health and the prevention of issues like osteoporosis and malnutrition.

Symptom Management: Dietary changes can help ease typical symptoms of biliary cholangitis, such as weariness, itching, and stomach pain. Avoiding foods that cause itching or pain, as well as adopting anti-inflammatory meals, can help offer relief and enhance quality of life.

Weight Management: Maintaining a healthy weight is critical for people with biliary cholangitis since excess weight can aggravate liver inflammation and increase the risk of complications. A well-balanced diet paired with frequent physical activity can aid in weight management and enhance overall health results.

Complication Prevention: By eating a diet customised to the demands of biliary cholangitis, people can lower their chance of developing cirrhosis, osteoporosis, and malabsorption. Emphasising nutrient-dense meals and limiting processed foods, alcohol, and saturated fats can help reduce these risks.

Choosing a diet that promotes liver function, controls bile flow, provides nutritional balance, manages symptoms, maintains a healthy weight, and prevents complications is critical for properly controlling biliary cholangitis. Working collaboratively with healthcare providers and nutritionists to create a personalised dietary plan is critical for improving outcomes and quality of life for people with this illness.

CHAPTER 2: OVERVIEW OF THE BILIARY CHOLANGITIS DIET:

Individuals with biliary cholangitis should follow a diet that promotes liver function, regulates bile flow, manages symptoms, and prevents complications. It emphasises nutrient-dense meals that are easy on the liver and enhance general health.

Key Nutritional Considerations:

Liver Support: Eat antioxidant-rich foods including fruits, vegetables, and whole grains to help your liver function and minimise inflammation.

Bile Flow Regulation: Eat foods high in soluble fibre, such as oats, beans, and legumes, to help control bile flow and reduce bile accumulation in the liver.

Nutritional Balance: To avoid nutritional deficiencies and promote general health, consume a balanced diet rich in protein, vitamins, minerals, and vital fatty acids.

Foods To Avoid:

High-Fat meals: Limit your consumption of saturated fats, fried meals, and fatty meats, since they might aggravate liver inflammation and reduce bile flow.

Processed meals: Avoid processed meals that contain additives, preservatives, and refined sugars, since they can strain the liver and exacerbate symptoms.

Alcohol: Alcohol can harm the liver and impair liver function in people with biliary cholangitis. It is critical to refrain from or restrict alcohol use when under medical care.

Foods To Include:

Fruits and Vegetables: Include a range of colourful fruits and vegetables, such as berries, leafy greens, and cruciferous vegetables, for antioxidant and anti-inflammatory benefits.

Whole Grains: Choose whole grains such as brown rice, quinoa, and whole wheat bread to give fibre and important nutrients without taxing the liver.

Lean Proteins: Choose lean protein sources including poultry, fish, tofu, and lentils, which supply vital amino acids without adding fat.

Importance of Hydration

Staying hydrated is critical for people with biliary cholangitis since it helps with liver function, digestion, and prevents problems like dehydration and constipation. Aim to drink lots of water throughout the day and avoid sugary and caffeinated beverages, which can dehydrate the body. Herbal teas, infused water, and electrolyte-rich drinks can also help with hydration and general health.

Individuals suffering with biliary cholangitis can enhance their quality of life by adhering to these dietary advice. It is critical to collaborate with healthcare specialists and nutritionists to create a personalised food plan that addresses individual needs and preferences.

CHAPTER 2: BREAKFAST DELIGHTS

Keto Sausage Egg Cups

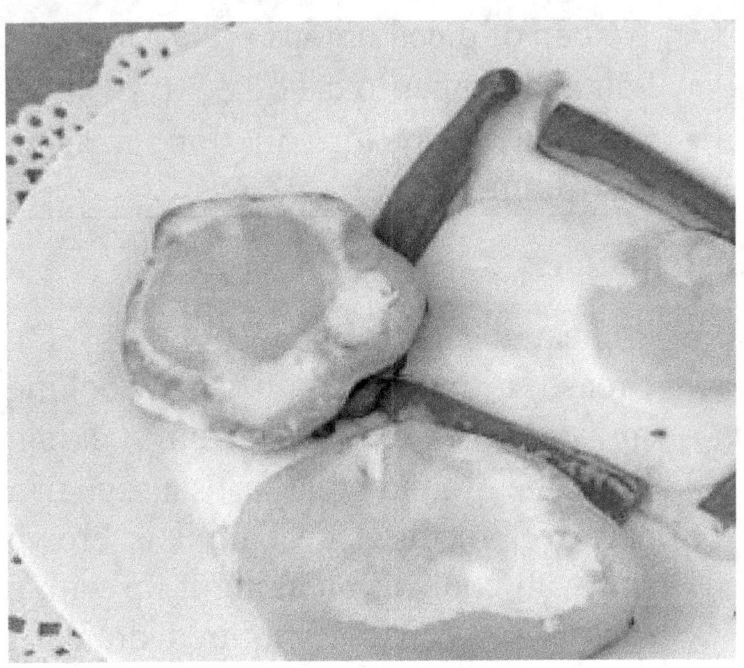

Ingredients:

- 6 big eggs
- 8 ounces of ground breakfast sausage (choose a low-carb option)
- 1/2 of cup shredded cheese (cheddar, mozzarella, or your preferred cheese)
- 1/4 cup of diced bell peppers
- 1/4 cup of diced onions
- Salt and pepper to taste
- Cooking spray or oil for greasing muffin tin

Instructions:

- Preheat the oven to 350°F (175° C). Grease a muffin tray with cooking spray or oil to keep them from sticking.
- Cook the ground breakfast sausage in a pan over medium heat until is brown and well cooked, breaking it up with a spatula as it cooks. If required, drain off any surplus fat.
- Crack the eggs into a mixing basin and beat them until thoroughly mixed. Season with salt and pepper to taste.

- Combine the cooked sausage, shredded cheese, chopped bell peppers, and diced onions with the beaten eggs until equally distributed.
- Pour the egg mixture into each muffin cup, filling it approximately 3/4 full.
- Bake in the preheated oven for 20-25 minutes, or until the egg cups are firm and gently brown.
- Remove from the oven and let the egg cups cool for a few minutes before carefully removing them from the muffin pan.
- Serve warm and enjoy!

Nutritional Value (per approximate serving):

Calories: 150 kcal

Total Fat: 11g

Saturated Fat: 4g

Trans Fat: 0g

Cholesterol: 195mg

Sodium: 270mg

Total Carbohydrates: 2g

Dietary Fibre: 0g

Sugars: 1g

Protein: 12g

Notes

Your

Observation

Blueberry Compote Oatmeal

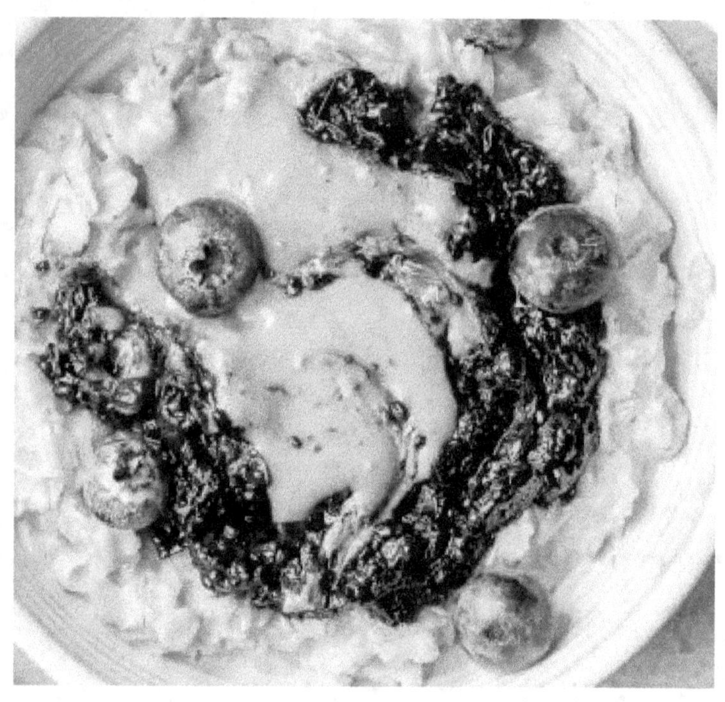

Ingredients:

- 1 cup of rolled oats
- 2 cups of water or your preferred milk
- 1 cup of fresh or frozen blueberries
- 2 tablespoons of maple syrup or honey
- 1 tablespoon of lemon juice
- 1/2 teaspoon vanilla extract
- Pinch of salt
- Optional toppings: sliced almonds, shredded coconut, additional fresh blueberries

Instructions:

- In a small saucepan, put together the blueberries, maple syrup or honey, lemon juice, vanilla essence, and a touch of salt.
- Bring to a simmer over medium heat, stirring periodically.
- When the blueberries begin to soften and release their juices, reduce the heat to low and let the compote to simmer

for approximately 5-7 minutes, or until slightly thickened.

- While the compote simmers, make the muesli. In a separate pot, heat the water or milk until it boils.
- Stir in the rolled oats and turn the heat down to low. Cook the muesli according to package directions, stirring periodically, until creamy and soft.
- When the muesli is done, take it off the fire and let it sit for a minute or two to thicken.
- Divide the muesli into serving dishes and top each with a liberal tablespoon of blueberry compote.
- If preferred, top with more fresh blueberries, sliced almonds, or shredded coconut.
- Serve the warm blueberry compote muesli and enjoy!

Nutritional Value (per approximate serving):

Calories: 250-300

Total Fat: 3-5g

Saturated Fat: 0.5-1g

Trans Fat: 0g

Cholesterol: 0mg

Sodium: 50-100mg

Total Carbohydrates: 50-60g

Dietary Fibre: 7-9g

Sugars: 20-25g

Protein: 5-7g

Notes

Your

Observation

Dandelion Greens Sauté

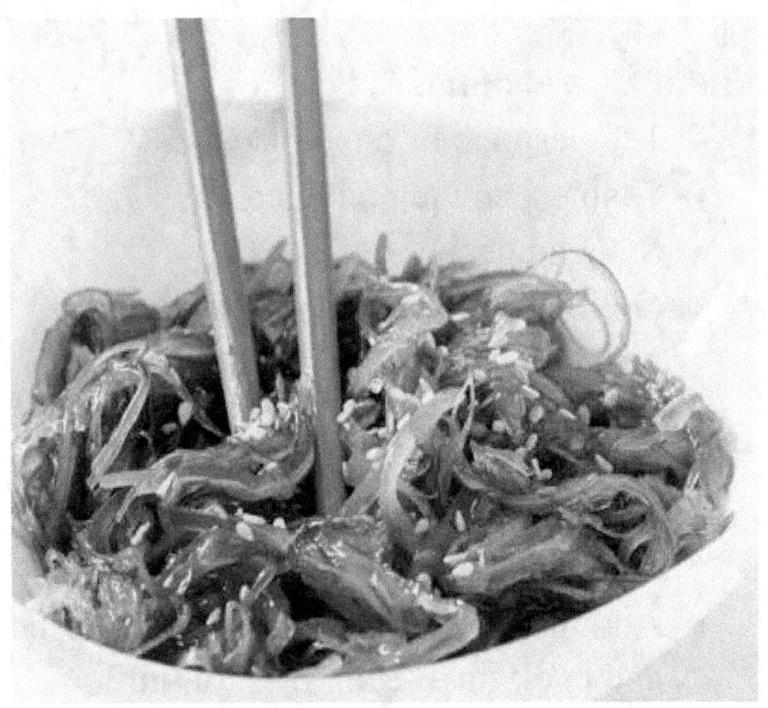

Ingredients:

- 1 bunch dandelion greens, washed and cut
- 2 cloves of minced garlic
- 1 tablespoon of olive oil
- 1 tablespoon lemon juice
- Salt and pepper to taste
- Optional: Red pepper flakes for added heat

Instructions:

- In a large saucepan, heat olive oil over medium heat.
- Add the minced garlic to the saucepan and cook for 1-2 minutes, or until fragrant.
- Add the chopped dandelion greens to the saucepan. Cook, stirring periodically, for 3-4 minutes, or until the greens wilt.

- Drizzle lemon juice over the greens, then simmer for another 2-3 minutes, or until tender.
- Season with salt, pepper, and (if using) red pepper flakes to taste.
- Remove the pan from the heat and place the dandelion greens on a serving dish.
- Serve hot as a healthful side dish or eat as a light and tasty dinner by itself.

Nutritional Value (per approximate serving):

Calories: 60

Total Fat: 4g

Saturated Fat: 0.5g

Trans Fat: 0g

Cholesterol: 0mg

Sodium: 120mg

Total Carbohydrates: 6g

Dietary Fibre: 4g

Sugars: 0g

Protein: 2g

Notes

Your

Observation

EAT HEALTHY AND BE HAPPY

CHAPTER 3: APPETIZERS FOR OPTIMAL DIGESTION

Avocado and Tomato Bruschetta

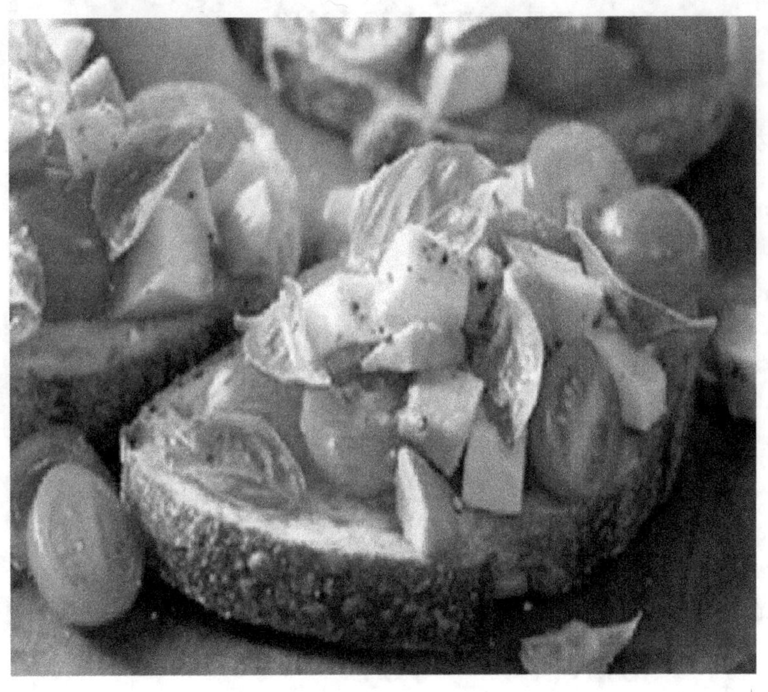

- 1 ripe avocado, chopped
- 1 cup of cherry tomatoes, diced
- 2 cloves of minced garlic
- 2 tablespoons of fresh basil, chopped
- 1 tablespoon of balsamic vinegar
- 1 tablespoon of extra virgin olive oil
- Salt and pepper to taste
- 1 baguette, sliced diagonally
- Optional: Balsamic glaze for drizzling

Instructions:

- In an average-sized mixing bowl, add the diced avocado, cherry tomatoes, minced garlic, fresh basil, balsamic vinegar, and extra virgin olive oil.
- Gently mix the ingredients until completely blended.
- Season the avocado and tomato combination with salt and pepper as desired.
- Preheat a grill pan or skillet to medium heat.

- Lightly coat both sides of each baguette slice with olive oil.
- Place the baguette slices in a hot grill pan or skillet. Toast each side until golden brown and crispy, about 1-2 minutes each side.
- Remove the toasted baguette slices from the grill pan or skillet and place on a serving plate.
- Spread the avocado and tomato mixture liberally on each toasted bread piece.
- Optional: Drizzle balsamic glaze over the avocado and tomato bruschetta to enhance flavour and appearance.
- Serve immediately as a tasty appetiser or small dinner.

Nutritional Value (per approximate serving):

Calories: 150

Total Fat: 8g

Saturated Fat: 1g

Trans Fat: 0g

Cholesterol: 0mg

Sodium: 150mg

Total Carbohydrates: 17g

Dietary Fibre: 3g

Sugars: 2g

Protein: 3g

Notes

Your

Observation

Cucumber Rolls with Hummus

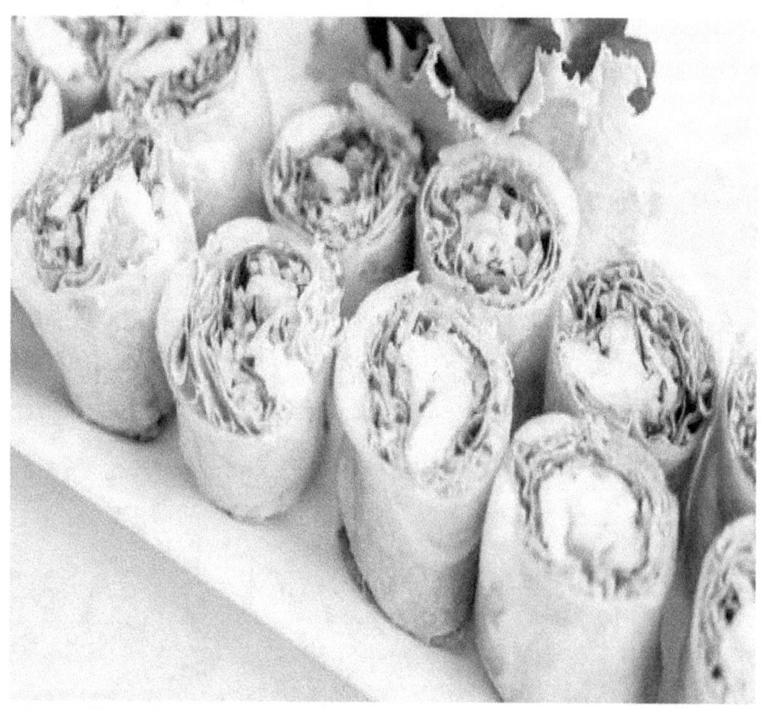

Ingredients:

- 1 big cucumber
- 1/2 cup of hummus (purchased or homemade)
- 1/4 cup of diced red bell pepper
- 1/4 cup of diced cucumber (from the same cucumber used for rolling)
- 1/4 cup of shredded carrots
- 1/4 cup of chopped fresh parsley or cilantro
- Salt and pepper to taste

Instructions:

- Use a vegetable peeler to finely slice the cucumber lengthwise into long strips. You can discard the first and last slices if they are largely peel.
- Place the cucumber strips flat on a clean surface.
- Spread a thin coating of hummus on each cucumber strip, leaving a little border on one side.

- Evenly spread the diced red bell pepper, diced cucumber, shredded carrots, and chopped fresh parsley or cilantro on the hummus-covered side of each cucumber strip.
- Sprinkle the vegetable filling with salt and pepper to taste.
- Starting from the filled side, gently coil each cucumber strip into a tight spiral.
- If necessary, use toothpicks to secure the rolls together.
- Place the cucumber rolls on a serving plate and serve immediately as a cool and healthful appetiser or snack.

Nutritional Value (per approximate serving):

Calories: 60

Total Fat: 3g

Saturated Fat: 0g

Trans Fat: 0g

Cholesterol: 0mg

Sodium: 150mg

Total Carbohydrates: 7g

Dietary Fibre: 2g

Sugars: 2g

Protein: 2g

Notes

Your

Observation

Beetroot and Walnut Dip

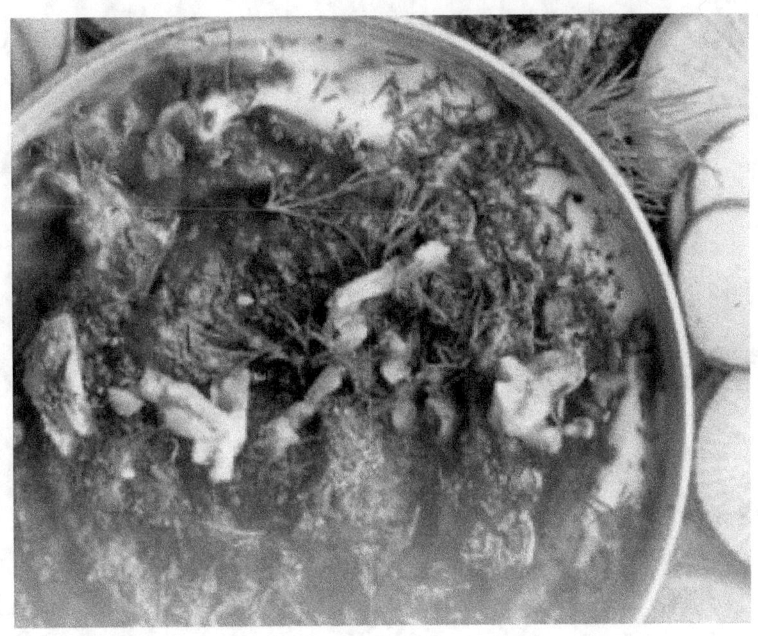

Ingredients:

- 2 average-sized beetroots, roasted and peeled
- 1/2 cup of walnuts
- 2 cloves of minced garlic
- 2 tablespoons of lemon juice
- 2 tablespoons of extra virgin olive oil
- 1 tablespoon of tahini
- Salt and pepper to taste
- Optional: Chopped fresh parsley or dill for garnish
- Optional: Toasted sesame seeds for garnish

Instructions:

- Preheat the oven to 400 °F (200 °C).
- Wrap each beetroot separately in aluminium foil and lay on a baking pan.
- Roast the beetroots in a preheated oven for 45-60 minutes, or until fork-tender.

- Remove the beetroots from the oven
  and allow to cool slightly before
  peeling off the skins. Discard the peels
  and cut the roasted beetroots into bits.
- In a food processor or blender, mix the
  roasted beets, walnuts, minced garlic,
  lemon juice, extra virgin olive oil, and
  tahini.
- Blend the ingredients until smooth and
  creamy, scraping down the edges of
  the bowl as necessary.
- Season the beetroot and walnut dip
  with salt and pepper as desired. Adjust
  the seasoning as needed.
- Transfer the dip to a serving bowl and
  top with chopped fresh parsley or dill
  and, if preferred, toasted sesame seeds.
- Serve the beetroot and walnut dip
  alongside your favourite crackers,
  breadsticks, or vegetable crudites.

Nutritional Value (per approximate serving):

Calories: 120

Total Fat: 10g

Saturated Fat: 1g

Trans Fat: 0g

Cholesterol: 0mg

Sodium: 60mg

Total Carbohydrates: 6g

Dietary Fibre: 2g

Sugars: 3g

Protein: 2g

Notes

Your

Observation

STAY

HEALTHY

CHAPTER 4: NOURISHING SOUPS AND SALADS

Healthy Chicken Noodle Soup

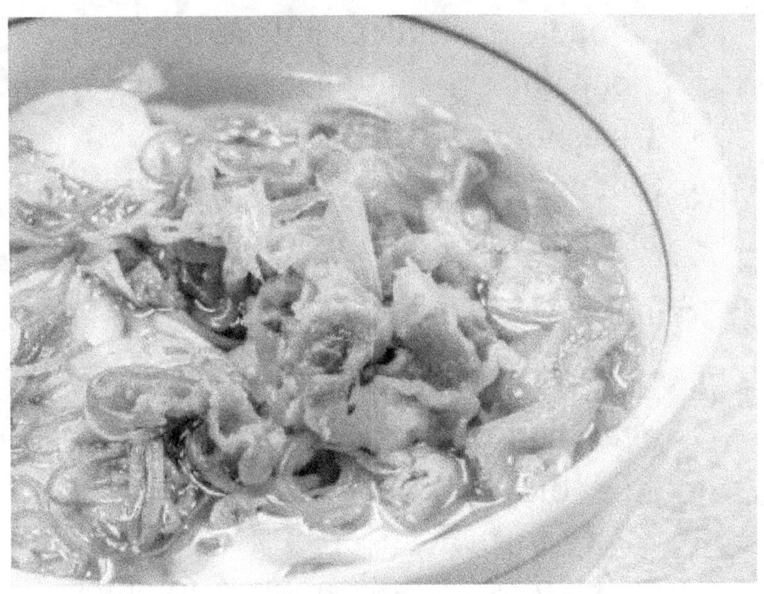

- 1 tablespoon of olive oil
- 1 onion, diced
- 2 carrots, sliced
- 2 celery stalks, sliced
- 2 cloves of minced garlic
- 6 cups of chicken broth
- 2 boneless, skinless chicken breasts
- 2 cups of egg noodles
- 1 teaspoon of dried thyme
- Salt and pepper to taste
- Fresh parsley, chopped, for garnish

Instructions:

- In a large saucepan, heat the olive oil over medium heat.
- Add the chopped onion, carrots, and celery to the saucepan. Sauté until the vegetables are soft, about 5 minutes.
- Add minced garlic to the saucepan and sauté for an additional 1-2 minutes, or until fragrant.

- Pour in the chicken broth and bring to a boil.
- Once the stock has boiled, add the boneless, skinless chicken breasts to the pot. Reduce the heat to low, cover, and simmer for 20-25 minutes, or until the chicken is fully cooked and tender.
- Remove the chicken breasts from the saucepan and place them on a chopping board. Using two forks, shred the chicken into bite-sized pieces.
- Return the shredded chicken to the pot. Add the egg noodles and dried thyme to the saucepan. Simmer for another 8-10 minutes, or until the noodles are cooked to your preferred doneness.
- Season the soup with salt and pepper, to taste.
- Ladle the healing chicken noodle soup into dishes and top with freshly chopped parsley.
- Serve hot and enjoy this cosy and nourishing soup.

Nutritional Value (per approximate serving):

Calories: 250

Total Fat: 6g

Saturated Fat: 1g

Trans Fat: 0g

Cholesterol: 60mg

Sodium: 800mg

Total Carbohydrates: 20g

Dietary Fibre: 2g

Sugars: 3g

Protein: 25g

Notes

Your

Observation

Springtime Salad with Chicken and Berries

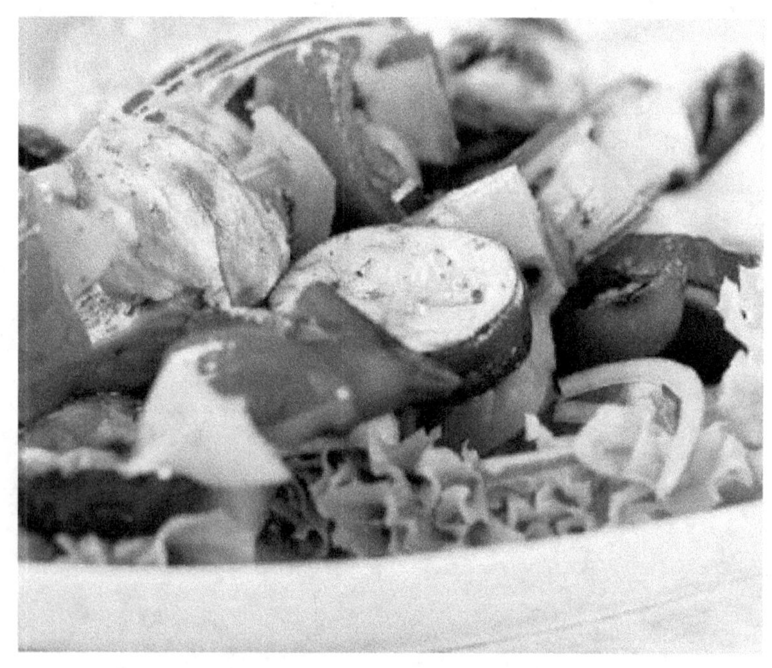

Ingredients:

- 2 boneless, skinless chicken breasts
- Salt and pepper to taste
- 6 cups of mixed salad greens (such as spinach, arugula, and lettuce)
- 1 cup of strawberries, hulled and chopped
- 1/2 cup of blueberries
- 1/4 cup of sliced almonds, toasted
- 1/4 cup of crumbled feta cheese
- 1/4 cup of balsamic vinaigrette dressing

Instructions:

- Season the chicken breasts with salt and pepper on both sides.
- Preheat a grill pan or skillet to medium-high heat. Cook the chicken breasts for 6-7 minutes on each side, or until well cooked and no longer pink in the centre. Remove from the heat and

allow it rest for a few minutes before slicing.

- While the chicken cooks, prepare the salad ingredients. In a large salad bowl, toss together the mixed salad greens, cut strawberries, blueberries, toasted almonds, and crumbled feta.
- After the chicken has rested, cut it into thin slices.
- Add the cut chicken to the salad bowl.
- Drizzle the balsamic vinaigrette dressing on the salad.
- Toss lightly to incorporate, making sure that the salad items are evenly coated with the dressing.
- Divide the spring salad with chicken and berries between serving dishes.
- Serve immediately as a light and refreshing lunch suitable for spring parties or picnics.

Nutritional Value (per approximate serving):

Calories: 350

Total Fat: 16g

Saturated Fat: 3g

Trans Fat: 0g

Cholesterol: 80mg

Sodium: 400mg

Total Carbohydrates: 18g

Dietary Fibre: 5g

Sugars: 9g

Protein: 32g

Notes

Your

Observation

Roasted Cauliflower & Potato Curry Soup

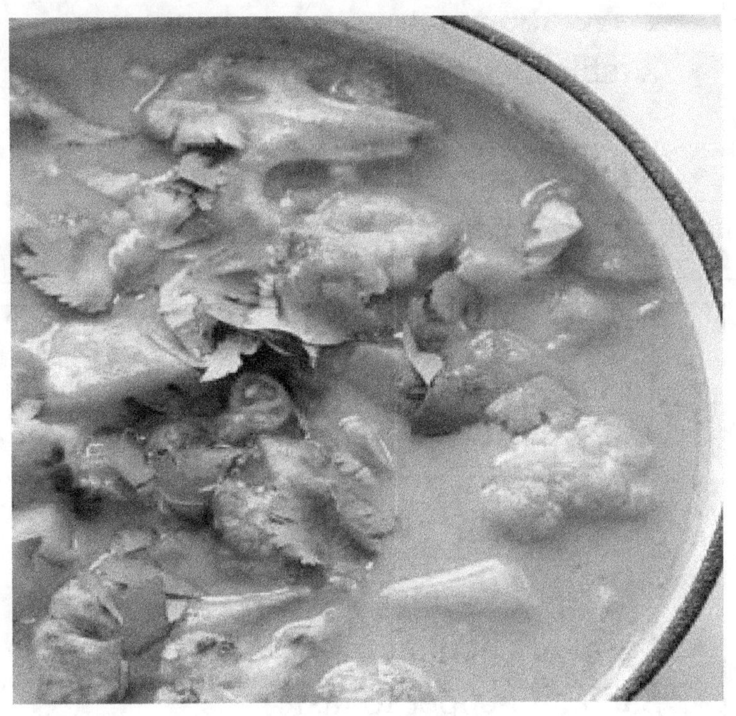

Ingredients:

For Roasting:

- 1 average cauliflower, cut into florets
- 2 average potatoes, peeled and diced
- 2 tablespoons of olive oil
- 1 teaspoon of curry powder
- Salt and pepper to taste

For Soup:

- Roasted cauliflower and potatoes
- 1 onion, chopped
- 2 cloves of minced garlic
- 1 tablespoon of grated fresh ginger
- 1 tablespoon of curry powder
- 4 cups of vegetable broth
- 1 cup of coconut milk
- Salt and pepper to taste
- Fresh cilantro, chopped, for garnish

Instructions:

For Roasting:

- Preheat the oven to 400 °F (200 °C).

- In a large mixing basin, combine the cauliflower florets and diced potatoes with the olive oil, curry powder, salt, and pepper until equally covered.
- Place the seasoned vegetables in a single layer on a baking sheet.
- Roast the cauliflower and potatoes in a preheated oven for 25-30 minutes, or until soft and golden brown.
- Remove the roasted vegetables from the oven and put them aside.

For Soup:

- In a large saucepan, heat 1 tablespoon of olive oil over medium heat.
- Sauté the chopped onion in the saucepan for about 5 minutes, or until transparent.
- Add the minced garlic, grated ginger, and curry powder to the saucepan. Cook for a further 2 minutes, stirring regularly.
- Place the roasted cauliflower and potatoes in the saucepan, followed by the vegetable broth.

- Bring the soup to a boil, then decrease the heat and simmer for 15-20 minutes to allow the flavours to combine.
- Use an immersion blender to purée the soup until it is smooth and creamy. Alternatively, transfer the soup to a blender in stages, blending until smooth before returning to the pot.
- Stir in the coconut milk and cook for another 5 minutes.
- Season with salt and pepper to taste.
- Ladle the roasted cauliflower and potato curry soup into serving dishes.
- Garnish with chopped fresh cilantro before serving.

Nutritional Value (per approximate serving):

Calories: 250

Total Fat: 15g

Saturated Fat: 9g

Trans Fat: 0g

Cholesterol: 0mg

Sodium: 600mg

Total Carbohydrates: 25g

Dietary Fibre: 5g

Sugars: 5g

Protein: 5g

Notes

Your

Observation

CHAPTER 5: SATISFYING MAIN DISHES

Baked Salmon with Dill Sauce

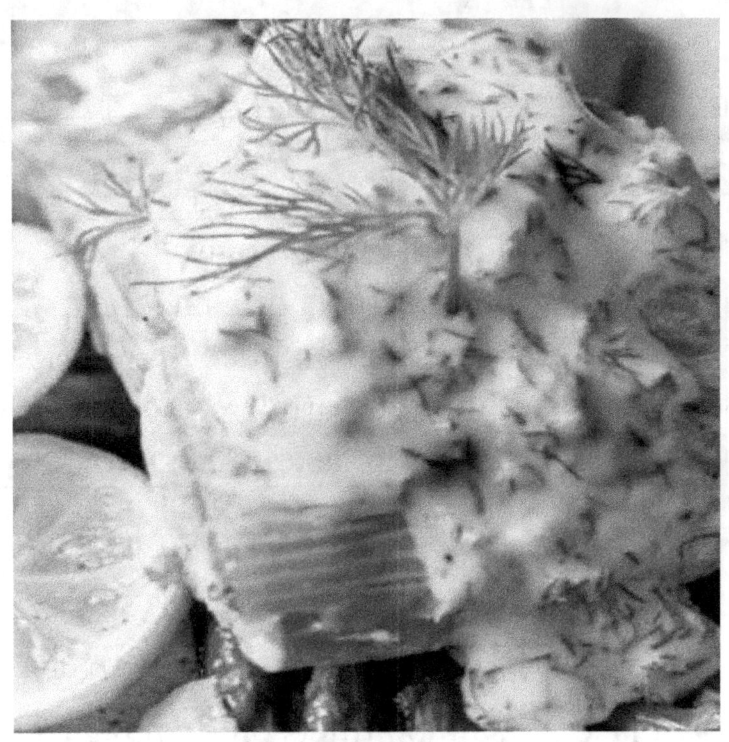

Ingredients:

For the Baked Salmon:

- 4 salmon fillets (about 6 ounces each)
- 2 tablespoons of olive oil
- Salt and pepper to taste
- Lemon slices for garnish

For the Dill Sauce:

- 1/2 cup of plain Greek yogurt
- 2 tablespoons of fresh dill, chopped
- 1 tablespoon of lemon juice
- 1 clove of minced garlic
- Salt and pepper to taste

Instructions:

For the Baked Salmon:

- Preheat the oven to 400 °F (200 °C).
- Place the salmon fillets on a baking pan covered with parchment or aluminium foil.

- Drizzle olive oil over the salmon fillets and season with salt and pepper.
- To enhance flavour, place a lemon slice on top of each salmon fillet.
- Bake in the preheated oven for 12-15 minutes, or until the salmon is fully cooked and readily flaked with a fork.

For the dill sauce:

- In a small mixing bowl, add Greek yoghurt, fresh dill, lemon juice, minced garlic, salt, and pepper. Mix thoroughly until all items are integrated.
- Taste and adjust seasoning to your liking.

Assembly:

- When the salmon is done, take it from the oven and transfer the fillets to serving plates.
- Spread the dill sauce liberally over each salmon fillet.
- If preferred, garnish with more fresh dill and lemon slices.

- Serve the baked salmon with dill sauce immediately, along with your favourite side dishes such roasted vegetables or steamed rice.

Nutritional Value (per approximate serving):

Calories: 300

Total Fat: 17g

Saturated Fat: 3g

Trans Fat: 0g

Cholesterol: 80mg

Sodium: 250mg

Total Carbohydrates: 3g

Dietary Fibre: 0g

Sugars: 1g

Protein: 33g

Notes

Your

Observation

Turkey and Vegetable Stir-Fry

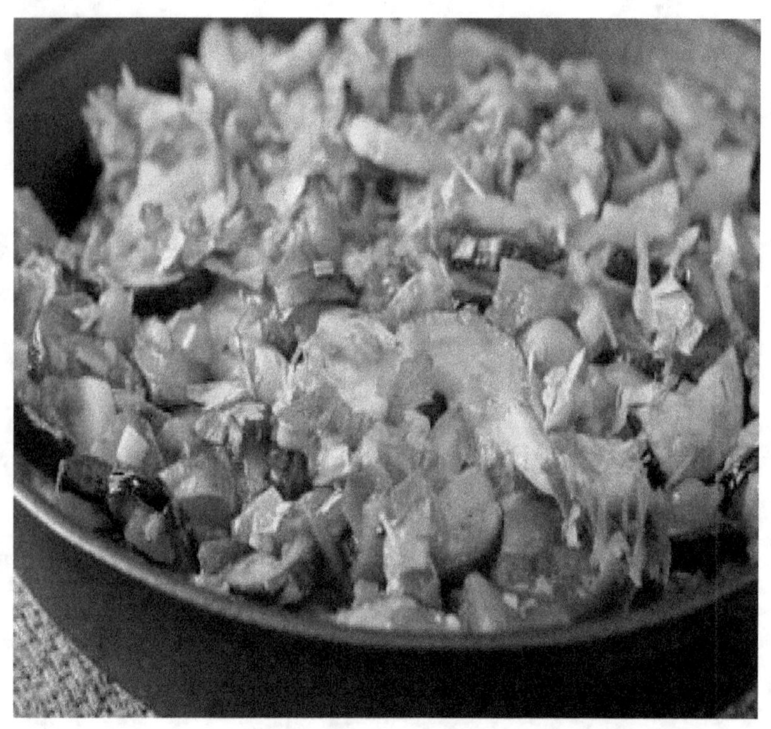

- 1 lb (450g) turkey breast, thinly sliced
- 2 tablespoons of soy sauce
- 1 tablespoon of oyster sauce
- 1 tablespoon of hoisin sauce
- 1 tablespoon of sesame oil
- 2 tablespoons of vegetable oil
- 2 cloves of minced garlic
- 1 teaspoon of minced ginger
- 1 onion, finely sliced
- 2 bell peppers (any colour), finely sliced
- 1 cup of broccoli florets
- 1 cup of snow peas, trimmed
- Salt and pepper to taste
- Cooked rice or noodles for serving
- Optional garnish: sliced green onions, sesame seeds

Instructions:

- In a small bowl, combine the soy sauce, oyster sauce, and hoisin sauce. Set aside.
- Heat the sesame and vegetable oils in a large pan or wok over medium-high heat.
- Cook the minced garlic and ginger in the pan for approximately 30 seconds, or until fragrant.
- Stir-fry the thinly sliced turkey breast for 2-3 minutes, or until well done.
- Remove the cooked turkey from the skillet and put it aside.
- Add a little more oil to the skillet if necessary, followed by the sliced onion, bell peppers, broccoli florets, and snow peas.
- Stir fry the veggies for 4-5 minutes, or until soft and crisp.
- Return the cooked turkey to the pan alongside the vegetables.

- Pour the sauce mixture onto the turkey and vegetables in the pan.
- Stir carefully to evenly coat everything with the sauce.
- Cook for a further 1-2 minutes, or until the sauce is thoroughly cooked and well mixed.
- Season with salt and pepper to taste.
- Serve the turkey and vegetable stir-fry hot with prepared rice or noodles.
- Garnish with chopped green onions and sesame seeds if preferred.
- Enjoy this tasty and healthful turkey and vegetable stir-fry!

Nutritional Value (per approximate serving):

Calories: 350-400

Total Fat: 15-20g

Saturated Fat: 2-4g

Trans Fat: 0g

Cholesterol: 60-80mg

Sodium: 700-900mg

Total Carbohydrates: 20-30g

Dietary Fibre: 4-6g

Sugars: 6-9g

Protein: 25-35g

Notes

Your
Observation

Lentil and Sweet Potato Shepherd's Pie

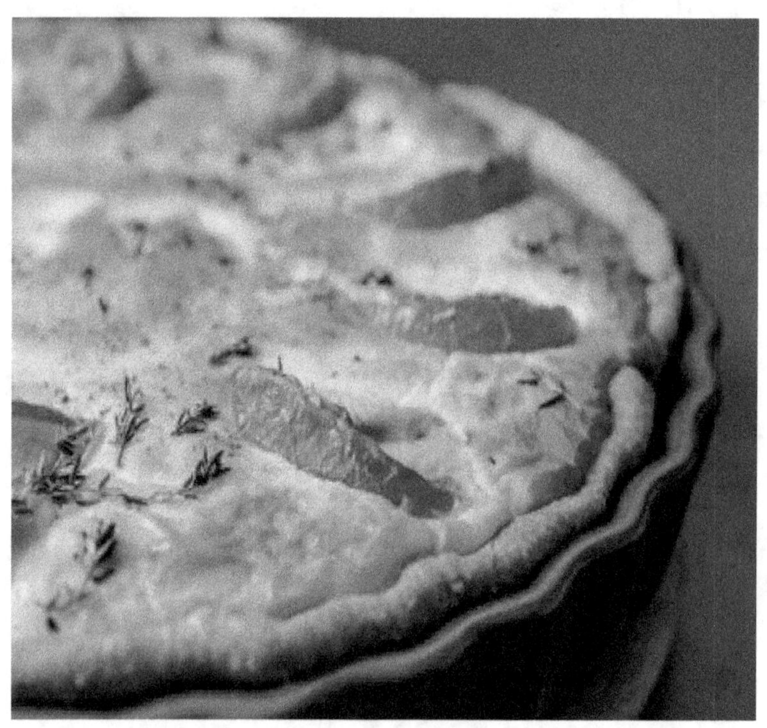

Ingredients:

For the Filling:

- 1 cup of dry green or brown lentils, rinsed
- 2 cups of vegetable broth
- 1 tablespoon of olive oil
- 1 onion, chopped
- 2 cloves of minced garlic
- 2 carrots, diced
- 2 celery stalks, diced
- 1 bell pepper, diced
- 1 cup of frozen peas
- 1 teaspoon of dried thyme
- 1 teaspoon of dried rosemary
- Salt and pepper to taste

For the Sweet Potato Topping:

- 2 big sweet potatoes, peeled and diced
- 2 tablespoons of butter or olive oil
- 1/4 cup of milk or vegetable broth (optional)

- Salt and pepper to taste

Instructions:

For the Filling:

- In an average saucepan, mix the rinsed lentils with the vegetable broth. Bring to a boil, then lower to a simmer for 20-25 minutes, or until the lentils are soft and the majority of the liquid has been absorbed. Drain the extra liquid and set it aside.
- In a large saucepan, heat the olive oil over medium heat. Sauté chopped onion and minced garlic until softened and aromatic, about 3-4 minutes.
- Add the chopped carrots, celery, and bell pepper to the saucepan. Cook for another 5-6 minutes, until the vegetables are soft.
- Add the cooked lentils, frozen peas, dried thyme, rosemary, salt, and pepper. Cook for another 2-3 minutes,

until everything is fully mixed and cooked through. Season to taste.

For the sweet potato topping:

- Bring a saucepan of water to a boil before adding the diced sweet potatoes. Cook the sweet potatoes for 10-15 minutes, or until fork-tender.
- Drain the cooked sweet potatoes and place them in a mixing basin.
- In a mixing dish, combine the sweet potatoes and butter or olive oil. Mash until smooth and creamy. If required, add milk or vegetable broth to reach the appropriate consistency. Season with salt and pepper to taste.

Assembly:

- Preheat the oven to 375°F (190° C).
- Transfer the lentil and veggie filling to a baking dish and distribute evenly.
- Spread the mashed sweet potatoes over the filling, covering the entire surface.

- Place the baking dish in the preheated oven for 25-30 minutes, or until the sweet potato topping is gently brown and the mixture is bubbling around the edges.
- Remove from the oven and allow it cool for a few minutes before serving.
- Serve the lentil and sweet potato shepherd's pie hot, topped with fresh herbs as desired.
- Enjoy your satisfying and nutritious lunch!

Nutritional Value (per approximate serving):

Calories: 300-350

Total Fat: 6-8g

Saturated Fat: 2-3g

Trans Fat: 0g

Cholesterol: 0mg

Sodium: 500-600mg

Total Carbohydrates: 50-60g

Dietary Fibre: 10-12g

Sugars: 10-12g

Protein: 12-15g

Notes

Your

Observation

CHAPTER 6: SIDE DISHES AND SNACKS

Roasted Eggplant with Miso and Sesame Seeds

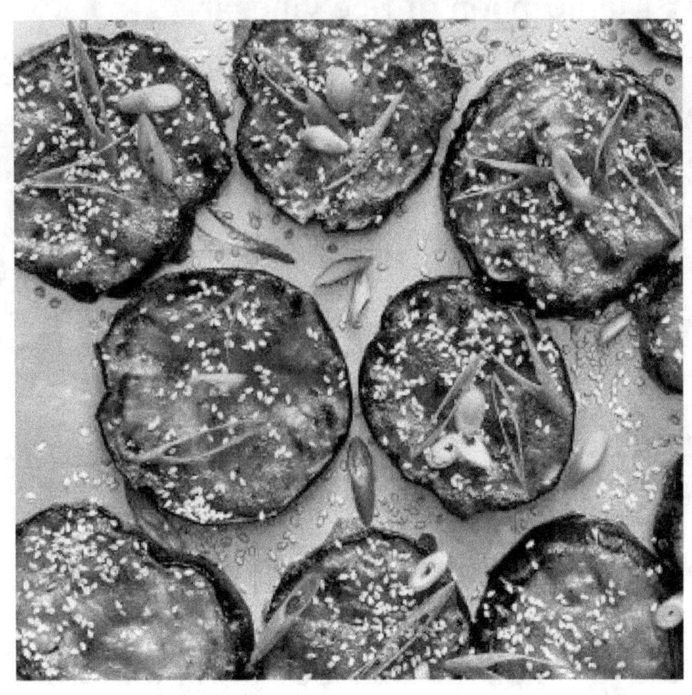

- 2 average-sized eggplants
- 2 tablespoons of white miso paste
- 2 tablespoons of sesame oil
- 1 tablespoon of soy sauce or tamari (for gluten-free option)
- 1 tablespoon of rice vinegar
- 1 tablespoon of maple syrup
- 2 cloves minced garlic
- 1 tablespoon of sesame seeds
- Green onions, thinly sliced (for garnish)
- Fresh cilantro leaves (for garnish)
- Cooked rice or quinoa (optional, for serving)

Instructions:

- Preheat the oven to 400 °F (200 °C).
- Wash the eggplants and cut them into circles or wedges about 1/2 inch thick.
- In a small mixing bowl, combine the miso paste, sesame oil, soy sauce or tamari, rice vinegar, maple syrup, and chopped garlic to prepare the marinade.

- Arrange the eggplant slices in a single layer on a baking sheet coated with parchment paper.
- Brush the eggplant slices thoroughly with the miso marinade, ensuring that they are equally coated.
- Sprinkle sesame seeds over the aubergine slices and gently press them into the marinade.
- Roast the aubergine in a preheated oven for 20-25 minutes, or until soft and caramelised, flipping once halfway through.
- When the aubergine is perfectly roasted, take it from the oven and place on a serving tray.
- Garnish with finely sliced green onions and fresh cilantro.
- If preferred, serve the roasted aubergine over cooked rice or quinoa. Enjoy!

Nutritional Value (per approximate serving):

Calories: 180-200

Total Fat: 10-12g

Saturated Fat: 1-2g

Trans Fat: 0g

Cholesterol: 0mg

Sodium: 400-500mg

Total Carbohydrates: 20-25g

Dietary Fibre: 6-8g

Sugars: 10-12g

Protein: 4-6g

Notes

Your

Observation

Crispy Baked Zucchini Fries

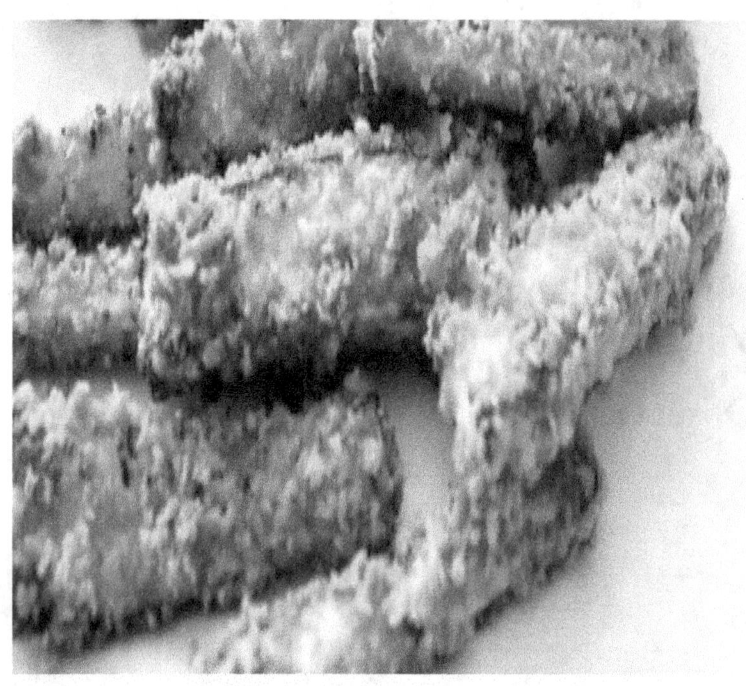

Ingredients:

- 2 average zucchinis
- 1/2 cup of all-purpose flour
- 2 big eggs, beaten
- 1 cup of breadcrumbs (preferably regular)
- 1/4 cup of grated Parmesan cheese
- 1 teaspoon of garlic powder
- 1 teaspoon of paprika
- 1/2 teaspoon of salt
- Cooking spray or olive oil

Instructions:

- Preheat the oven to 425°F (220°C). Line a baking sheet with parchment paper or aluminium foil, then gently coat with cooking spray or olive oil.
- Wash the zucchinis and cut them into long strips like French fries.
- In a shallow basin or plate, put together the breadcrumbs, grated Parmesan

cheese, garlic powder, paprika, and salt. Mix thoroughly.

- Put the flour in another shallow basin, then the beaten eggs in a third shallow bowl.
- Dredge each zucchini strip in flour and shake off the excess.
- Dip the floured zucchini strip in the beaten eggs, covering fully.
- Then, carefully press the breadcrumb mixture onto the zucchini strip to ensure it adheres.
- Place the oiled zucchini strip on the prepared baking sheet. Repeat for the remaining zucchini strips.
- Once all of the zucchini strips have been coated and placed on the baking sheet, gently spray them with cooking spray or drizzle with olive oil for added crispiness.
- Bake in the preheated oven for 20-25 minutes, turning halfway through, or

until the zucchini fries are golden brown and crispy.

- Remove from the oven and allow to cool slightly before serving.
- Serve the crispy baked zucchini fries hot with your preferred dipping sauce, such as marinara, ranch dressing or aioli.

Nutritional Value (per approximate serving):

Calories: 150

Total Fat: 5g

Saturated Fat: 1g

Trans Fat: 0g

Cholesterol: 60mg

Sodium: 350mg

Total Carbohydrates: 20g

Dietary Fibre: 2g

Sugars: 3g

Protein: 7g

Notes

Your

Observation

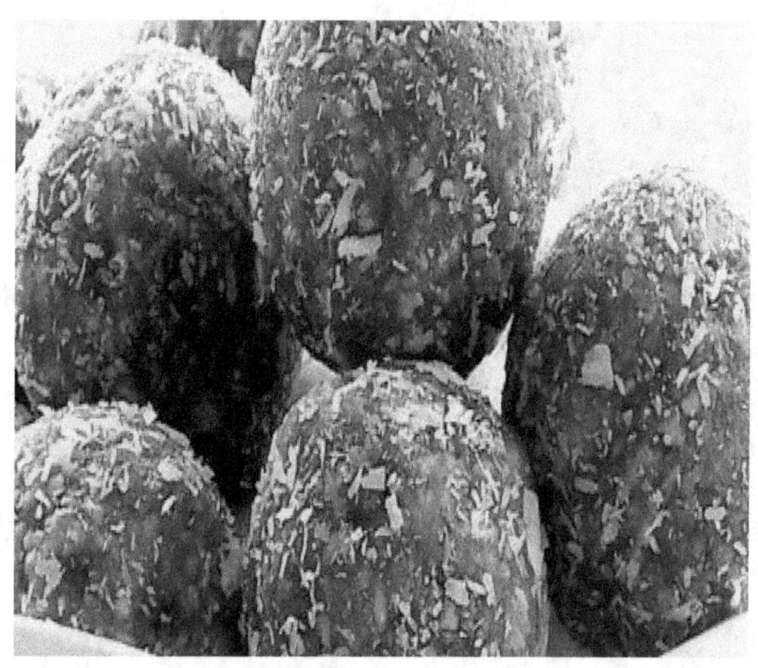

Ingredients:

- 1 cup of pitted dates
- 1 cup of almonds
- 2 tablespoons of cocoa powder
- 1 tablespoon of honey or maple syrup (optional)
- 1/2 teaspoon of vanilla extract
- Pinch of salt
- Desiccated coconut or chopped nuts for coating (optional)

Instructions:

- In a food processor, put together the pitted dates, almonds, cocoa powder, honey or maple syrup (if using), vanilla essence, and a sprinkle of salt.

- Pulse the ingredients until they are fully blended and have a sticky dough consistency. If the mixture is too dry, add a tablespoon of water at a time, until it comes together.

- When the mixture is finished, use a spoon or your hands to scoop out tiny bits and shape them into balls between your palms.
- If preferred, coat the energy balls with desiccated coconut or chopped almonds for an added layer of flavour and texture.
- Place the rolled energy balls on a baking sheet covered with parchment paper.
- Refrigerate the energy balls for at least 30 minutes until firm.
- Once cold, place the energy balls in an airtight container and refrigerate for up to two weeks.
- These almond and date energy balls are a nutritious and tasty snack for when you need a fast dose of energy!

Nutritional Value (per approximate serving):

Calories: 70-80

Total Fat: 3-4g

Saturated Fat: 0g

Trans Fat: 0g

Cholesterol: 0mg

Sodium: 0mg

Total Carbohydrates: 10-12g

Dietary Fibre: 2g

Sugars: 8-9g

Protein: 2g

Notes

Your

Observation

CHAPTER 7: DESSERT OPTIONS

Berry Chia Seed Pudding

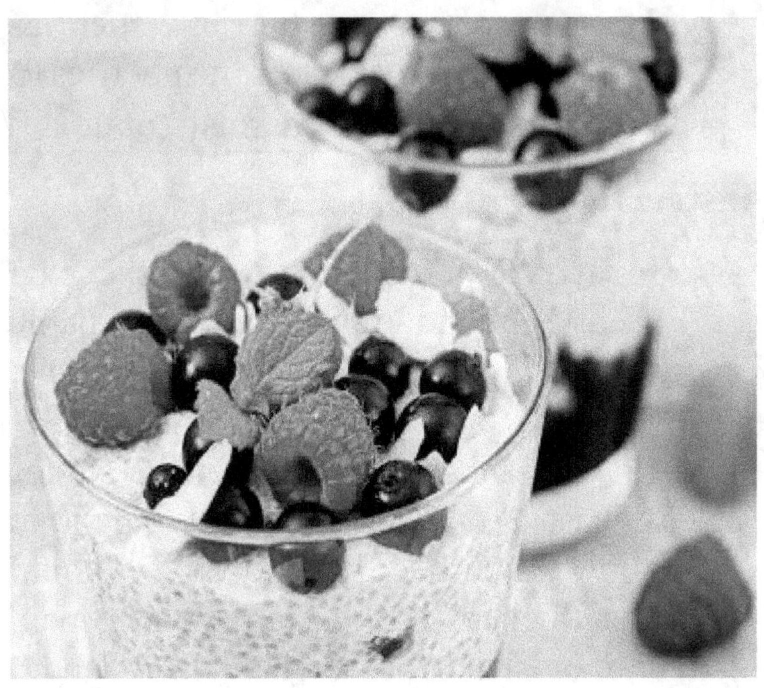

Ingredients:

- 1/4 cup of chia seeds
- 1 cup of unsweetened almond milk (or any preferred choice)
- 1 tablespoon of honey or maple syrup (optional, adjust to taste)
- 1/2 teaspoon of vanilla extract
- 1/2 cup of mixed berries (such as strawberries, blueberries, raspberries)
- Fresh mint leaves for garnish (optional)

Instructions:

- In a dish or container, mix the chia seeds, almond milk, honey or maple syrup (if using), and vanilla essence. Stir well to mix.
- Cover the dish or jar and refrigerate for at least 2 hours, preferably overnight, to allow the chia seeds to absorb the liquid and thicken to a custard consistency. Stir or shake occasionally throughout this time to avoid clumping.

- After the chia seed pudding has thickened, give it one more stir to break up any clumps.
- In serving glasses or bowls, top the chia seed pudding with the mixed berries.
- Garnish with fresh mint leaves if preferred.
- This delicious and nutritious berry chia seed pudding is perfect for breakfast, snacking or dessert! Serve chilled!

Nutritional Value (per approximate serving):

Calories: 150-200

Total Fat: 7-10g

Saturated Fat: 0.5-1g

Trans Fat: 0g

Cholesterol: 0mg

Sodium: 50-100mg

Total Carbohydrates: 20-25g

Dietary Fibre: 8-10g

Sugars: 8-12g

Protein: 5-7g

Notes

Your

Observation

Dark Chocolate Avocado Mousse

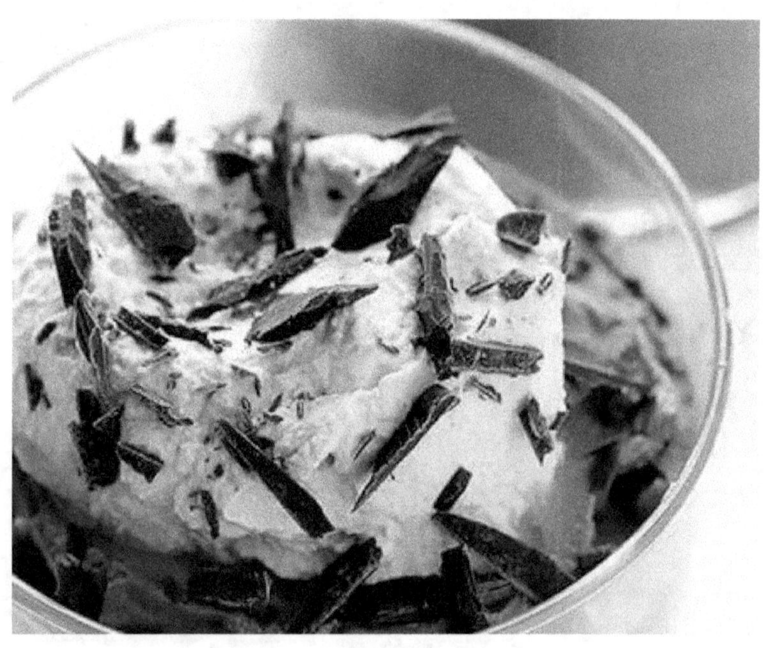

Ingredients:

- 2 ripe avocados
- 1/4 cup of unsweetened cocoa powder
- 1/4 cup of maple syrup or honey (adjust to taste)
- 1 teaspoon of vanilla extract
- Pinch of salt
- 1/4 cup of unsweetened almond milk or coconut milk
- Optional toppings: fresh berries, chopped nuts, shredded coconut

Instructions:

- Cut the avocados in halves, remove the pits, and transfer the flesh to a blender or food processor.
- Combine the cocoa powder, maple syrup or honey, vanilla extract, salt, and almond milk in a blender or food processor.
- Blend or process until the mixture is smooth and creamy, scraping down the

edges as required to ensure thorough mixing.

- Taste the mousse and adjust the sweetness or chocolate flavour as needed by adding additional maple syrup or cocoa powder.
- Once the mousse has reached the correct consistency and flavour, transfer it to serving dishes or glasses.
- Wrap the bowls or cups in plastic wrap and freeze for at least 30 minutes to firm up.
- Garnish the dark chocolate avocado mousse with fresh fruit, chopped nuts, or shredded coconut, if preferred.
- Enjoy this delicious and nutritious dessert when cold!

Nutritional Value (per approximate serving):

Calories: 200-250

Total Fat: 14-18g

Saturated Fat: 3-4g

Trans Fat: 0g

Cholesterol: 0mg

Sodium: 10-20mg

Total Carbohydrates: 24-30g

Dietary Fibre: 7-9g

Sugars: 14-18g

Protein: 3-4g

Notes

Your

Observation

Baked Apples with Cinnamon and Walnuts

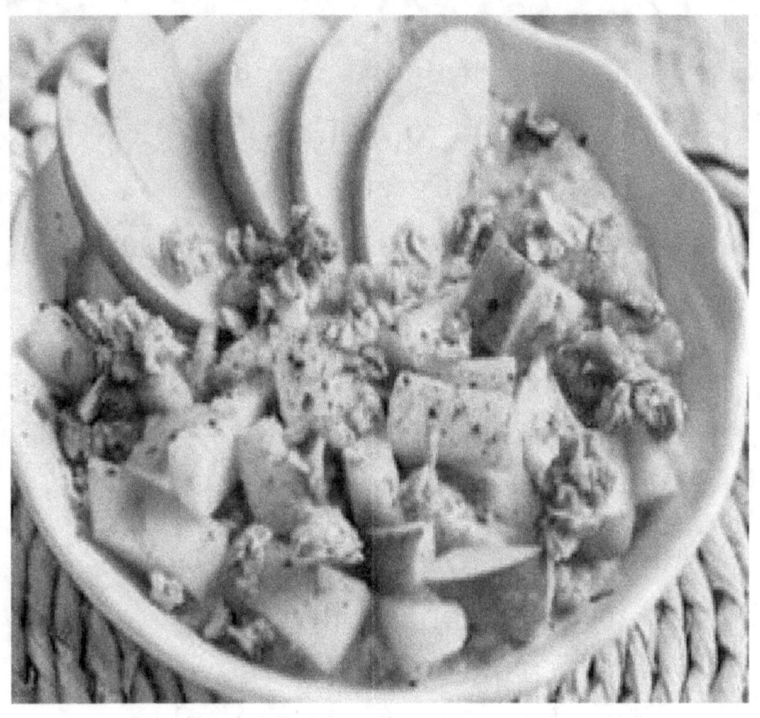

Ingredients:

- 4 big apples (such as Honey crisp or Granny Smith)
- 1/4 cup of walnuts, chopped
- 2 tablespoons of honey or maple syrup
- 1 teaspoon of ground cinnamon
- 1 tablespoon of unsalted butter, melted (optional)
- Vanilla ice cream or whipped cream for serving (optional)

Instructions:

- Preheat the oven to 375°F (190° C).
- Wash the apples, then blot them dry with a paper towel. Remove the cores from the apples using an apple corer or a tiny knife, leaving the bottoms intact.
- In a small bowl, blend the chopped walnuts, honey or maple syrup, and ground cinnamon until thoroughly incorporated.

- Stuff each cored apple with the walnut mixture, pushing it tightly in the centre.
- Place the packed apples in a baking dish, standing up.
- Drizzle melted butter over each filled apple, if desired.
- Cover the baking dish with aluminium foil and bake for 25-30 minutes, or until the apples can be poked with a fork.
- Remove the foil from the baking dish and bake for another 5-10 minutes, or until the apples' tops are softly golden brown.
- Remove the roasted apples from the oven and allow them cool slightly before serving.
- Serve the baked apples warm, with a scoop of vanilla ice cream or whipped cream on top.

Nutritional Value (per approximate serving):

Calories: 150-200

Total Fat: 7-10g

Saturated Fat: 1-2g

Trans Fat: 0g

Cholesterol: 0mg

Sodium: 0mg

Total Carbohydrates: 25-30g

Dietary Fibre: 4-6g

Sugars: 18-22g

Protein: 1-2g

Notes

Your

Observation

JUICING AND SMOOTHIES FOR BILIARY CHOLANGITIS

CHAPTER 8

Liver Lovin' Smoothie

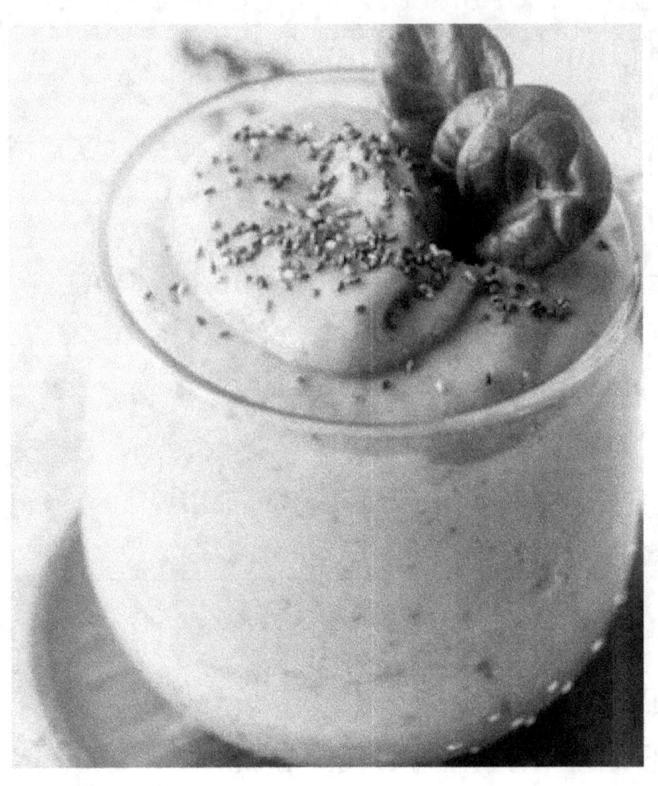

- 1 cup of spinach leaves, fresh
- 1 small beet, peeled and cut
- 1/2 cup of blueberries, fresh or frozen
- 1/2 inch of fresh ginger, peeled
- 1/2 lemon, juiced
- 1 tablespoon of chia seeds
- 1 tablespoon of flaxseed meal
- 1 cup unsweetened almond milk or coconut water
- Optional: 1 teaspoon honey or maple syrup for added sweetness
- Ice cubes (optional, for a colder smoothie)

Instructions:

- Put all of the ingredients in a blender.
- Blend till smooth and creamy, then add ice cubes if you like a cooler smoothie.
- Adjust the sweetness and sharpness of the smoothie by adding extra honey, maple syrup, or lemon juice as needed.

- Pour the smoothie into a glass after it has reached the appropriate consistency and flavour.
- Serve immediately and enjoy your Liver Lovin' smoothie as a pleasant and healthy method to promote liver health!

Nutritional Value (per approximate serving):

Calories: 150-200

Total Fat: 6-8g

Saturated Fat: 0.5-1g

Trans Fat: 0g

Cholesterol: 0mg

Sodium: 100-150mg

Total Carbohydrates: 20-25g

Dietary Fiber: 6-8g

Sugars: 10-15g

Protein: 4-6g

Notes

Your

Observation

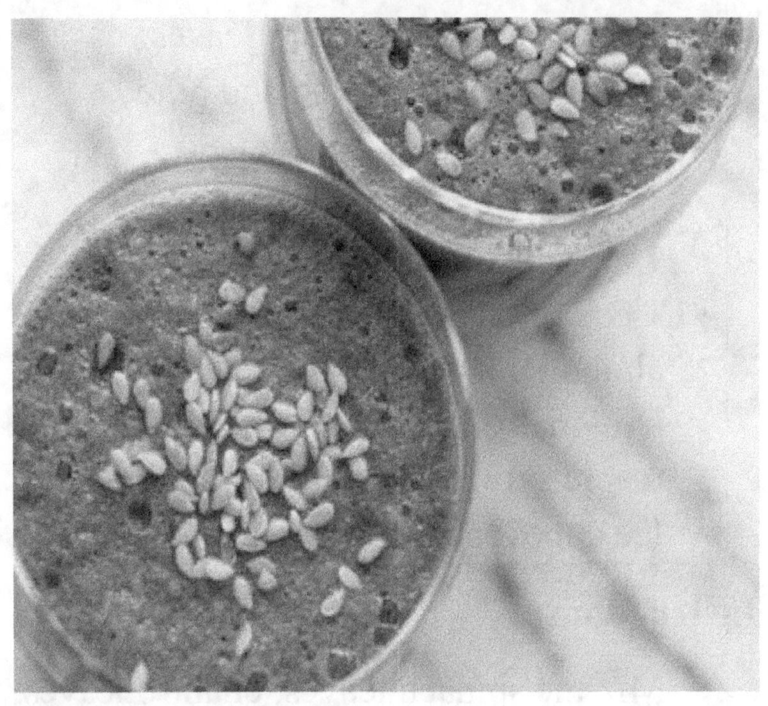

Ingredients:

- 1 cup of fresh spinach leaves
- 1/2 cup of fresh cilantro leaves
- 1 ripe avocado, peeled and pitted
- 1/2 cucumber, peeled and cut
- 1/2 lime, juiced
- 1 tablespoon of chia seeds
- 1 cup of unsweetened coconut water or almond milk
- Optional: 1 teaspoon of honey or maple syrup for added sweetness
- Ice cubes (optional, for a colder shake)

Instructions:

- Mix the spinach leaves, cilantro leaves, avocado, sliced cucumber, lime juice, chia seeds, and coconut or almond milk in a blender.
- Blend until smooth and creamy, then add ice cubes if you like a cooler shake.

- Adjust the sweetness and sharpness of the smoothie by adding extra honey, maple syrup, or lime juice as needed.
- Pour the shake into a glass after it has reached the required consistency and flavour.
- Serve immediately and enjoy your Green attractiveness Cilantro Shake as a pleasant and healthy method to promote overall health and attractiveness!

Nutritional Value (per approximate serving):

Calories: 200-250

Total Fat: 15-20g

Saturated Fat: 2-3g

Trans Fat: 0g

Cholesterol: 0mg

Sodium: 100-150mg

Total Carbohydrates: 20-25g

Dietary Fiber: 8-10g

Sugars: 5-8g

Protein: 4-6g

Notes

Your

Observation

Healthy "Shamrock" Shake

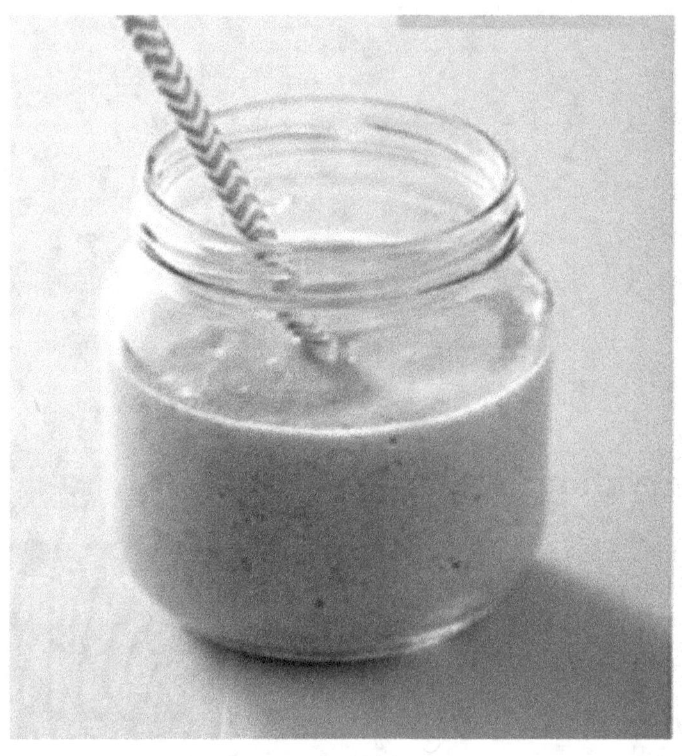

Ingredients:

- 1 ripe banana, frozen
- 1/2 cup of spinach leaves, fresh
- 1/2 cup of unsweetened almond milk (or any preferred choice)
- 1/4 of teaspoon peppermint extract
- 1/4 of teaspoon vanilla extract
- Optional: 1 tablespoon of honey or maple syrup for added sweetness
- Ice cubes (optional, for a colder shake)
- Whipped cream or Greek yogurt for topping (optional)
- Fresh mint leaves for garnish (optional)

Instructions:

- Blend together the frozen banana, spinach leaves, almond milk, peppermint extract, and vanilla extract.
- If desired, add honey or maple syrup to sweeten.

- Blend until smooth and creamy, then add ice cubes if you like a cooler shake.
- Taste the smoothie and adjust the sweetness or mint flavour as needed by adding additional sugar or peppermint extract.
- Pour the shake into a glass after it has reached the required consistency and flavour.
- If preferred, top the shake with whipped cream or Greek yoghurt for extra richness.
- Garnish with fresh mint leaves for a festive finish.
- Serve immediately and enjoy your green "Shamrock" smoothie as a pleasant and nutritious snack!

Nutritional Value (per approximate serving):

Calories: 120-150

Total Fat: 1-2g

Saturated Fat: 0g

Trans Fat: 0g

Cholesterol: 0mg

Sodium: 80-100mg

Total Carbohydrates: 25-30g

Dietary Fiber: 3-4g

Sugars: 15-20g

Protein: 2-3g

Notes

Your Observation

4-3-2-1 Green Smoothie

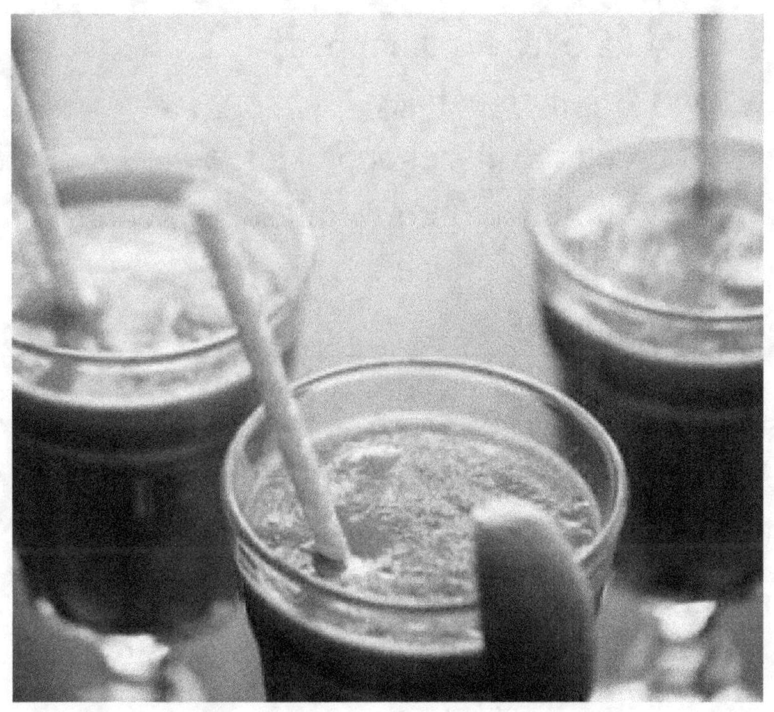

Ingredients:

- 4 kale leaves, chopped
- 1/3 bunch parsley
- 2 celery ribs, chopped large
- 1 apple, cut into wedges
- 1/2 lemon, juiced
- 2 cups of water

Instructions:

- Wash and prepare all of the ingredients as directed.
- In a blender, add kale leaves, parsley, celery ribs, apple wedges, lemon juice, and water.
- Blend until smooth, adjusting the consistency with extra water as needed.
- Taste the smoothie and modify the flavour as needed by adding extra lemon juice or honey.

- When the smoothie has reached the required consistency and flavour, pour it into glasses.
- Serve immediately and enjoy your delicious Kale and Parsley Green Smoothie!

Nutritional Value (per approximate serving):

Calories: 50-70

Total Fat: 0-1g

Saturated Fat: 0g

Trans Fat: 0g

Cholesterol: 0mg

Sodium: 30-50mg

Total Carbohydrates: 12-15g

Dietary Fibre: 4-6g

Sugars: 7-9g

Protein: 2-3g

Notes

Your

Observation

Bok Choy Green Smoothie

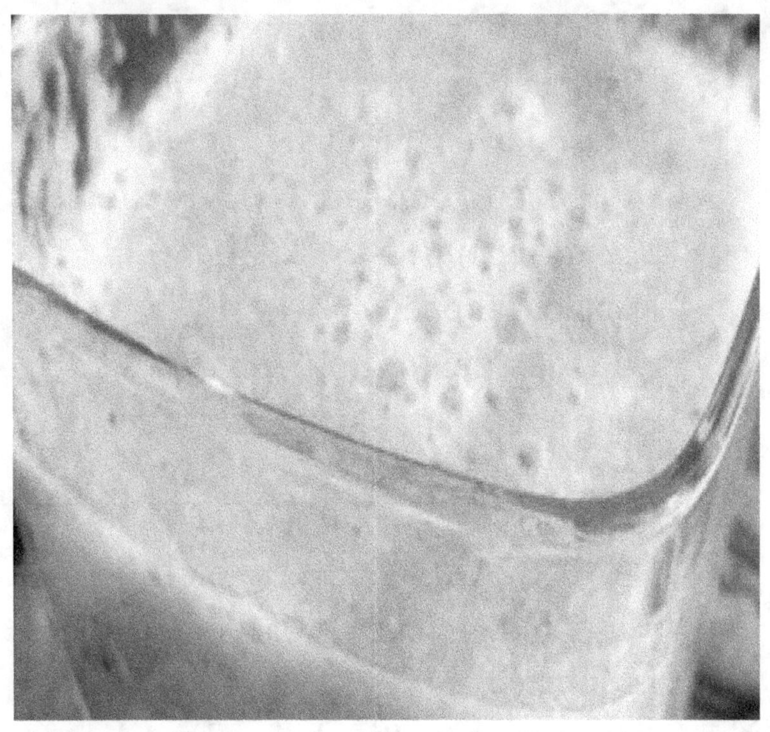

- 1-2 cups of bok choy leaves
- 1 whole English cucumber
- 10 parsley, basil, or mint leaves
- 1 teaspoon of spirulina (optional)
- 1 teaspoon of maca powder (optional)
- 2 pears, chopped
- 1 apple, chopped
- 1-2 inch of piece fresh ginger
- 2 cups of water, plus extra for desired consistency

Instructions:

- Wash and prepare all of the ingredients as directed.
- Add together the bok choy leaves, cucumber, parsley (or basil or mint) leaves, spirulina, maca powder, chopped pears, chopped apple, fresh ginger, and water.

- Blend until smooth, adding additional water as needed to get the desired consistency.
- Taste the smoothie and adjust the sweetness or flavour as needed by adding extra fruit or ginger.
- When the smoothie has reached the required consistency and flavour, pour it into glasses.
- Serve immediately and enjoy your healthy Bok Choy Green Smoothie!

Nutritional Value (per approximate serving):

Calories: 100-150

Total Fat: 1-2g

Saturated Fat: 0g

Trans Fat: 0g

Cholesterol: 0mg

Sodium: 20-30mg

Total Carbohydrates: 25-30g

Dietary Fibre: 6-8g

Sugars: 15-20g

Protein: 2-3g

Notes

Your

Observation

Golden Turmeric Latte Smoothie

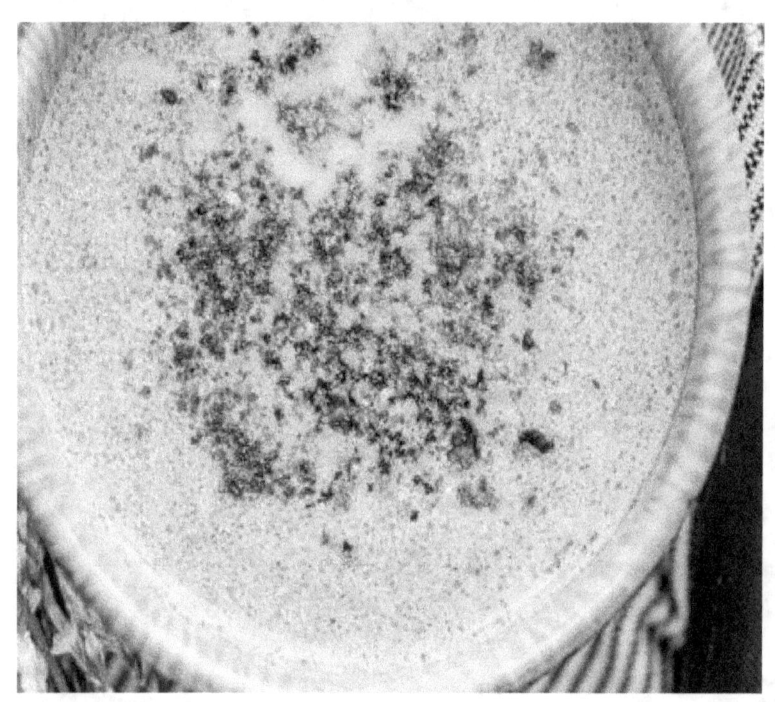

Ingredients:

- 1 ripe banana
- 1 cup of unsweetened almond milk or coconut milk
- 1 teaspoon of ground turmeric
- 1/2 teaspoon of ground cinnamon
- 1/4 teaspoon of ground ginger
- 1/8 teaspoon of ground black pepper
- 1 tablespoon of honey or maple syrup (optional, for sweetness)
- 1/2 teaspoon of vanilla extract
- Ice cubes (optional, for a colder smoothie)

Instructions:

- Peel the ripe banana and chop it into bits.
- Blend together the banana chunks, almond milk or coconut milk, ground turmeric, cinnamon, ginger, black

pepper, honey or maple syrup (if using), and vanilla essence.

- Blend until smooth and creamy.
- Taste the smoothie and adjust the sweetness or spice levels as needed by adding additional honey, maple syrup, turmeric, or spices.
- If you want a cooler smoothie, add ice cubes to the blender and process again until smooth.
- When the smoothie has reached the required consistency and flavour, pour it into glasses.
- Serve immediately and enjoy your Golden Turmeric Latte Smoothie as a tasty and nutritious treat!

Nutritional Value (per approximate serving):

Calories: 150-200

Total Fat: 2-3g

Saturated Fat: 0g

Trans Fat: 0g

Cholesterol: 0mg

Sodium: 100-150mg

Total Carbohydrates: 30-35g

Dietary Fibre: 3-5g

Sugars: 20-25g

Protein: 1-2g

Notes

Your

Observation

Dandelion Beetroot juice

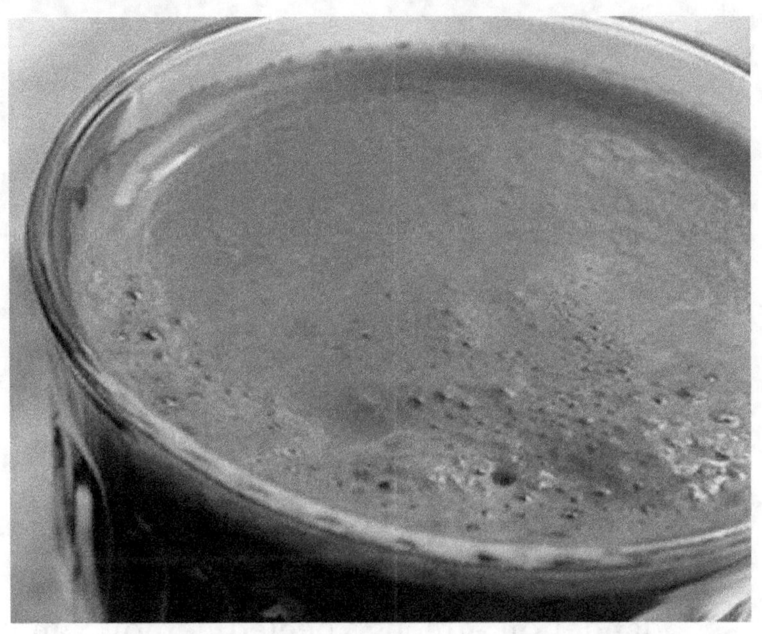

Ingredients:

- 2 big beets, peeled
- 2 apples
- 2 cups of packed dandelion greens
- 1 lemon, peeled
- 1 inch of fresh ginger root

Instructions:

- Wash and prepare all of the ingredients as directed.
- Cut the beets and apples into pieces that fit through the juicer chute.
- In a juicer, combine the beets, apples, dandelion greens, peeled lemon, and fresh ginger root.
- After juicing all of the ingredients, mix to blend the flavours.
- If preferred, strain the juice through a fine mesh screen or cheesecloth to eliminate any pulp.
- Pour some juice into a glass.

- Serve immediately and enjoy the delicious Dandelion Beetroot Juice.

Nutritional Value (per approximate serving):

Calories: 150-200

Total Fat: 1-2g

Saturated Fat: 0g

Trans Fat: 0g

Cholesterol: 0mg

Sodium: 100-150mg

Total Carbohydrates: 35-40g

Dietary Fibre: 8-10g

Sugars: 25-30g

Protein: 3-5g

Notes

Your

Observation

Blast of broccoli smoothie

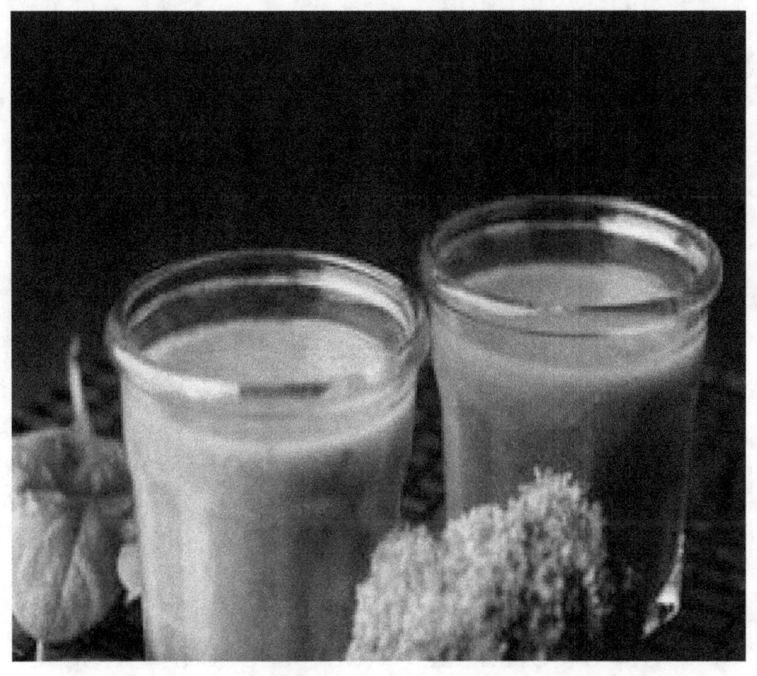

- 1 cup of broccoli florets
- 1 ripe banana
- 1/2 cup of pineapple chunks (fresh or frozen)
- 1/2 cup of spinach leaves
- 1 tablespoon of chia seeds
- 1 cup of unsweetened almond milk or coconut water
- Ice cubes (optional, for a colder smoothie)

Instructions:

- Wash and prepare all of the ingredients as directed.
- In a blender, add broccoli florets, banana, pineapple pieces, spinach leaves, chia seeds, and almond milk or coconut water.
- Blend until smooth and creamy, then add ice cubes if you like a cooler smoothie.

- Taste the smoothie and adjust the sweetness or flavour as needed by adding extra fruit or honey.
- When the smoothie has reached the required consistency and flavour, pour it into glasses.
- Serve immediately and enjoy your Blast of Broccoli Smoothie!

Nutritional Value (per approximate serving):

Calories: 150-200

Total Fat: 3-5g

Saturated Fat: 0.5-1g

Trans Fat: 0g

Cholesterol: 0mg

Sodium: 100-150mg

Total Carbohydrates: 30-35g

Dietary Fibre: 8-10g

Sugars: 15-20g

Protein: 3-5g

Notes

Your

Observation

Lemon-Lime Coconut Smoothie

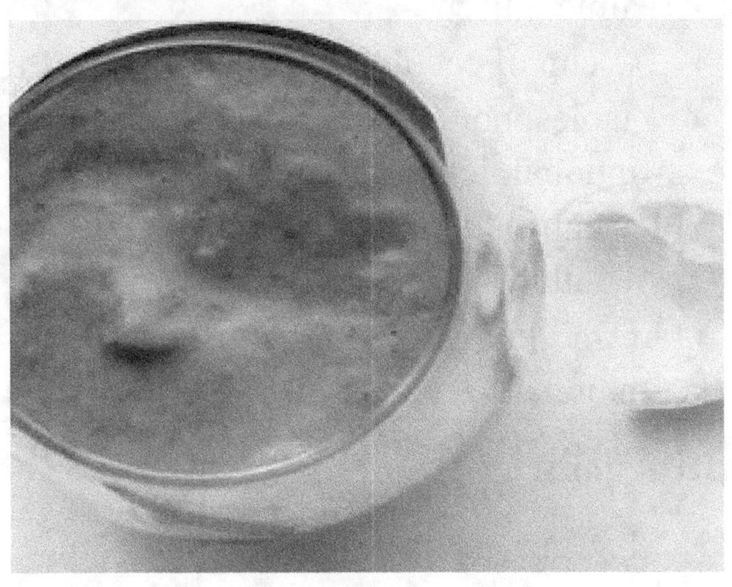

- 1 cup of coconut water
- 1 lemon, juiced
- 1 lime, juiced
- 1/2 cup of coconut milk
- 1 tablespoon of honey or maple syrup (optional, for sweetness)
- Ice cubes (optional, for a colder smoothie)
- Fresh mint leaves for garnish (optional)

Instructions:

- Mix the coconut water, lemon juice, lime juice, coconut milk, and honey or maple syrup (if preferred) in a blender.
- Blend until smooth and creamy.
- Taste the smoothie and adjust the sweetness or tartness as needed by adding more honey or lime juice.

- If you want a cooler smoothie, add ice cubes to the blender and process again until smooth.
- When the smoothie has reached the required consistency and flavour, pour it into glasses.
- Garnish with fresh mint leaves if preferred.
- Serve immediately and enjoy your delightful Lemon-Lime Coconut Smoothie.

Nutritional Value (per approximate serving):

Calories: 100-150

Total Fat: 5-7g

Saturated Fat: 4-5g

Trans Fat: 0g

Cholesterol: 0mg

Sodium: 20-30mg

Total Carbohydrates: 15-20g

Dietary Fibre: 1-2g

Sugars: 10-15g

Protein: 1-2g

Notes

Your

Observation

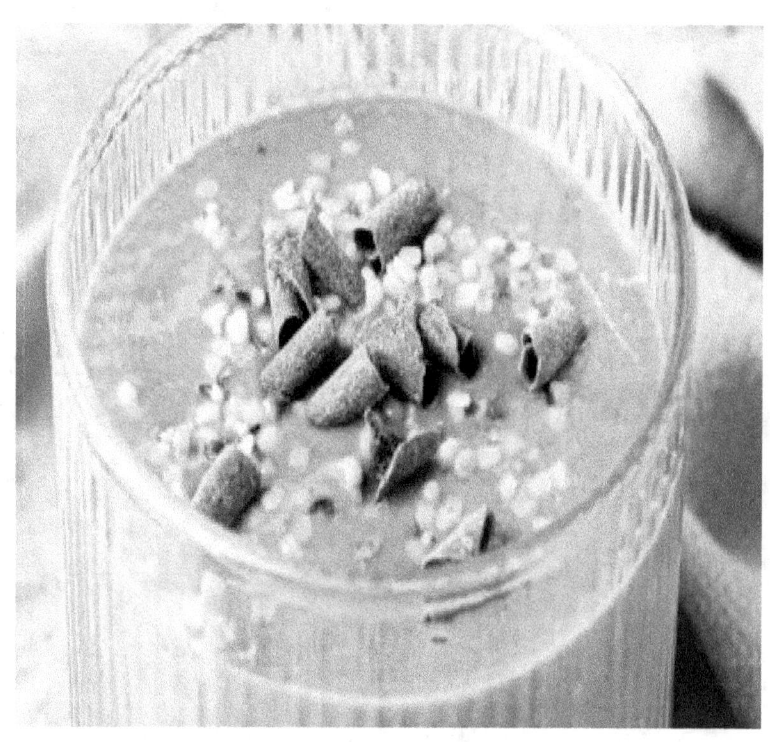

Ingredients:

- 1 ripe banana
- 1 tablespoon of unsweetened cocoa powder
- 1 tablespoon of almond butter
- 1 tablespoon of honey or maple syrup (optional, for sweetness)
- 1 cup of unsweetened almond milk or coconut milk
- Ice cubes (optional, for a colder smoothie)
- Chocolate chips or cocoa powder for garnish (optional)

Instructions:

- Peel the ripe banana and chop it into bits.
- In a blender, add banana chunks, unsweetened cocoa powder, almond butter, honey or maple syrup (if using), and almond or coconut milk.
- Blend until smooth and creamy.

- Taste the smoothie and adjust the sweetness as needed by adding additional honey or cocoa powder.
- If you want a cooler smoothie, add ice cubes to the blender and process again until smooth.
- When the smoothie has reached the required consistency and flavour, pour it into glasses.
- Garnish with chocolate chips or cocoa powder if desired.
- Serve immediately and enjoy your wonderful Banana Chocolate Smoothie!

Nutritional Value (per approximate serving):

Calories: 200-250

Total Fat: 8-10g

Saturated Fat: 1-2g

Trans Fat: 0g

Cholesterol: 0mg

Sodium: 50-100mg

Total Carbohydrates: 30-35g

Dietary Fibre: 4-6g

Sugars: 20-25g

Protein: 3-5g

Notes

Your

Observation

Green machine smoothie

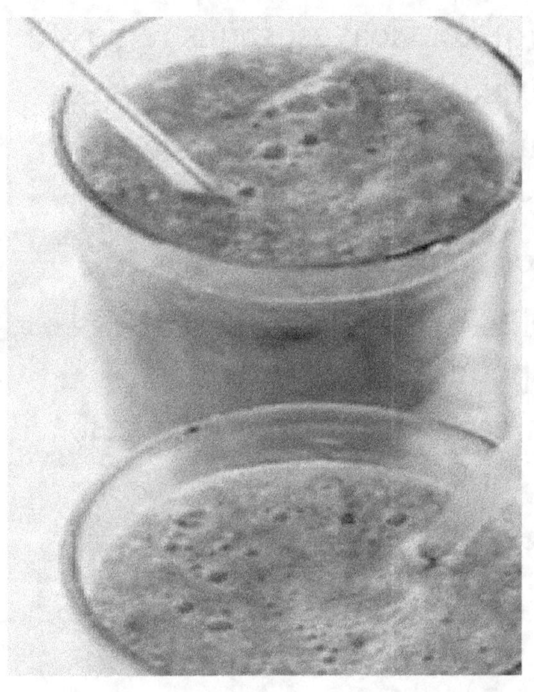

Ingredients:

- 1 cup of spinach leaves
- 1/2 cup of kale leaves, stems removed
- 1/2 ripe avocado
- 1/2 cucumber, peeled and chopped
- 1/2 green apple, cored and chopped
- 1/2 lemon, juiced
- 1 tablespoon of fresh ginger, grated
- 1 tablespoon of chia seeds
- 1 cup of coconut water or unsweetened almond milk
- Ice cubes (optional, for a colder smoothie)

Instructions:

- Wash and prepare all of the ingredients as directed.
- In a blender, add spinach, kale, avocado, cucumber, green apple, lemon juice, grated ginger, chia seeds, and coconut water or almond milk.

- Blend until smooth and creamy, then add ice cubes if you like a cooler smoothie.
- Taste the smoothie and modify the flavour as needed by adding extra lemon juice or ginger.
- Pour the smoothie into glasses once you have achieved the correct consistency and taste.
- Serve immediately and enjoy the delicious Green Machine Smoothie!

Nutritional Value (per approximate serving):

Calories: 150-200

Total Fat: 8-10g

Saturated Fat: 1-2g

Trans Fat: 0g

Cholesterol: 0mg

Sodium: 50-100mg

Total Carbohydrates: 20-25g

Dietary Fibre: 8-10g

Sugars: 8-10g

Protein: 4-6g

Green Detox Smoothie

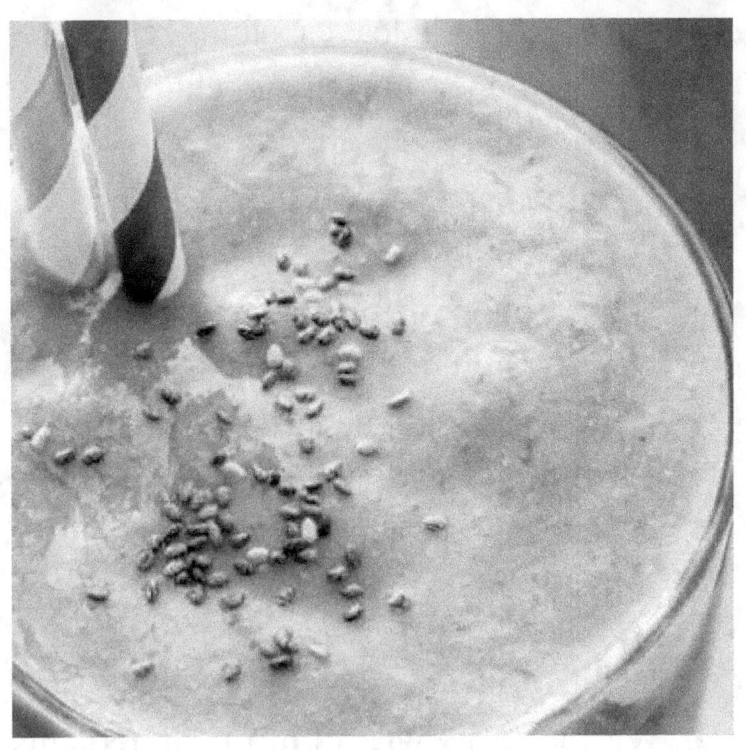

Ingredients:

- 1 cup of spinach leaves
- 1/2 cup of kale leaves, stems removed
- 1/2 cucumber, peeled and chopped
- 1 stalk celery, chopped
- 1/2 green apple, cored and chopped
- 1/2 lemon, juiced
- 1 tablespoon of fresh ginger, grated
- 1 tablespoon of chia seeds
- 1 cup of coconut water or unsweetened almond milk
- Ice cubes (optional, for a colder smoothie)

Instructions:

- Wash and prepare all of the ingredients as directed.
- In a blender, add spinach, kale, cucumber, celery, green apple, lemon juice, grated ginger, chia seeds, and coconut water or almond milk.

- Blend until smooth and creamy, then add ice cubes if you want a cooler smoothie.
- Taste the smoothie and modify the flavour as needed by adding extra lemon juice or ginger.
- Pour the smoothie into glasses once you have achieved the correct consistency and taste.
- Serve immediately and enjoy your revitalising Green Detox Smoothie!

Nutritional Value (per approximate serving):

Calories: 100-150

Total Fat: 3-5g

Saturated Fat: 0.5-1g

Trans Fat: 0g

Cholesterol: 0mg

Sodium: 50-100mg

Total Carbohydrates: 15-20g

Dietary Fibre: 6-8g

Sugars: 7-9g

Protein: 3-4g

Notes

____

____

____

____

____

____

Your

Observation

____

____

____

____

____

____

CHAPTER 9

Adapting recipes for special dietary needs

Gluten-free Options:

Substitute gluten-free grains like quinoa, rice, millet, or buckwheat for wheat-based cereals including barley, wheat, and rye.

Choose gluten-free flours such as almond flour, coconut flour, or gluten-free all-purpose flour for baking.

Choose gluten-free pasta made with rice, quinoa, or chickpeas.

Include naturally gluten-free foods including fruits, vegetables, legumes, nuts, seeds, and proteins like chicken, fish, and tofu.

Dairy-free Alternatives:

Replace dairy milk with almond milk, coconut milk, rice milk, oat milk, or soy milk.

Cook and bake with dairy-free margarine or coconut oil instead of butter.

Use dairy-free yoghurt prepared with coconut, almond, or soy milk.

Choose dairy-free cheese substitutes derived from almonds or soy.

Look for dairy-free creamers and whipped toppings prepared with coconut or almond milk.

Low-FODMAP Adjustments:

Select low-FODMAP fruits and vegetables including strawberries, blueberries, oranges, carrots, cucumbers, spinach, and bell peppers.

Reduce high-FODMAP vegetables such as onions, garlic, cauliflower, and mushrooms.

Choose gluten-free grains such as rice, quinoa, and oats instead of wheat-based items.

To avoid high-FODMAP dairy products, replace milk, yoghurt, and cheese with lactose-free or dairy-free alternatives.

Avoid some sweets, such as honey and agave syrup, and instead go for low-FODMAP alternatives like maple syrup or stevia.

Avoid high-FODMAP legumes such as beans and lentils, and instead use tofu or tempeh as plant-based protein sources.

To keep FODMAP levels low, flavour foods using garlic-infused oil rather than garlic cloves.

Limit your consumption of processed meals and snacks containing high-FODMAP components such as fructans, sorbitol, and mannitol.

Individuals with biliary cholangitis should see a healthcare physician or a qualified dietitian to develop a personalised diet plan that addresses their particular dietary needs and preferences while effectively treating their illness.

CHAPTER 10: 7 DAY MEAL PLAN

Day 1

Breakfast: Green smoothie (spinach, banana, almond milk, chia seeds)

Lunch: Cucumber rolls with Hummus

Dinner: Baked salmon with dill sauce

Day 2:

Breakfast: Blue berry compote oatmeal

Lunch: Avocado and tomato bruschetta

Dinner: Turkey and vegetable stir-fry

Day 3:

Breakfast: Dandelion Greens Sauté

Lunch: Roasted eggplant with miso and sesame seeds

Dinner: Lentil and sweet potato shepherd's pie

Day 4:

Breakfast: Keto Sausage Egg Cups

Lunch: Crispy baked zucchini fries

Dinner: Berry chia seed pudding

Day 5:

Breakfast: Roasted cauliflower and potato curry soup

Lunch: Beetroot and walnut dip

Dinner: Bok choy green smoothie

Day 6:

Breakfast: Healthy chicken noodle soup

Lunch: Almond and date energy balls

Dinner: Baked apples with cinnamon and walnuts

Day 7:

Breakfast: Avocado toast on gluten-free bread with cherry tomatoes

Lunch: Dark chocolate Avocado mousse

Dinner: Blast of broccoli smoothie

CHAPTER 11:
CONCLUSION

A biliary cholangitis cookbook might be a useful resource for people living with this ailment. It enables people to make good food choices that help ease symptoms and promote optimum liver function by providing tasty and nutritious recipes designed to enhance liver health and general well-being.

The cookbook tackles particular nutritional issues such as combining liver-friendly products, avoiding triggers that may worsen symptoms, and catering to dietary limitations such as gluten-free, dairy-free, and low-FODMAP alternatives. These dishes are intended to be both savoury and mild on the digestive system, allowing people with biliary cholangitis to have delicious meals without jeopardising their health.

Furthermore, the cookbook emphasises the value of a well-balanced and diversified diet high in fruits, vegetables, lean meats, whole grains, and healthy fats. These nutrient-dense meals provide critical vitamins, minerals, antioxidants, and fibre, which help the liver detoxify, decrease inflammation, and maintain general health.

Individuals who follow the recipes and directions described in the biliary cholangitis cookbook can take proactive actions to manage their disease and improve their quality of life. However, it is critical to note that dietary adjustments should be done in cooperation with a healthcare professional or certified dietitian to ensure they are appropriate for your specific requirements and medical recommendations.

In essence, a biliary cholangitis cookbook provides not just delectable dishes, but also practical advice and help for negotiating the challenges of nutritional control.

STAY HEALTHY!

Bonus

MEAL
PLANNER
DAILY
DATE
BREAKFAST
NOTES
LUNCH
SNACK
ITEMS LIST
DINNER

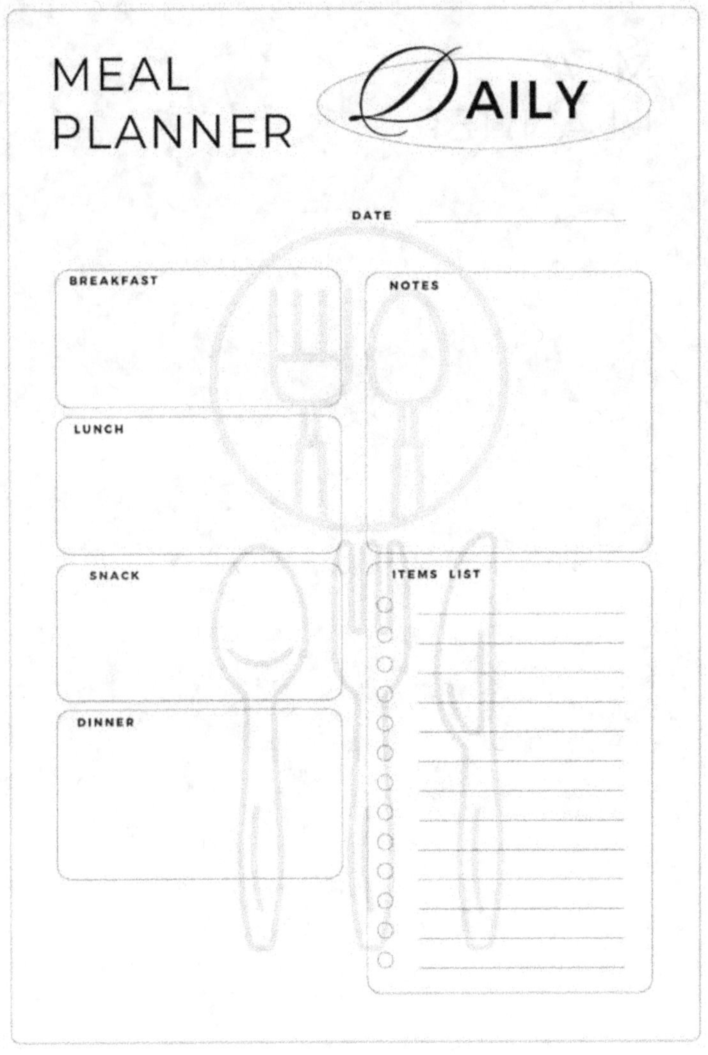

MEAL PLANNER

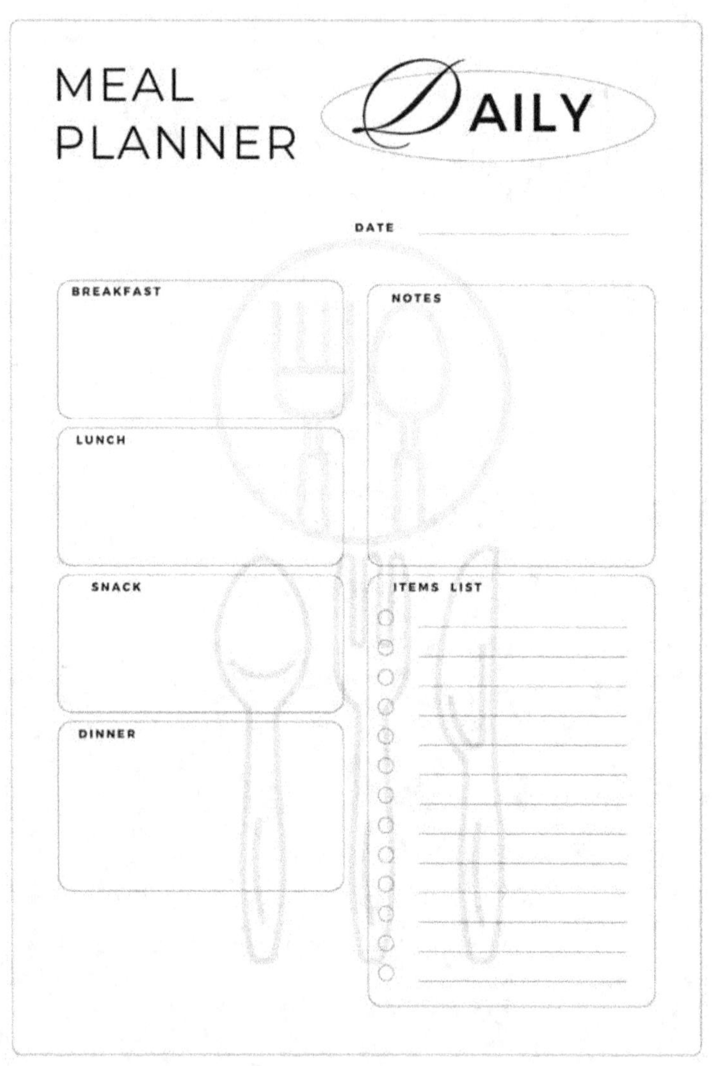

MEAL PLANNER

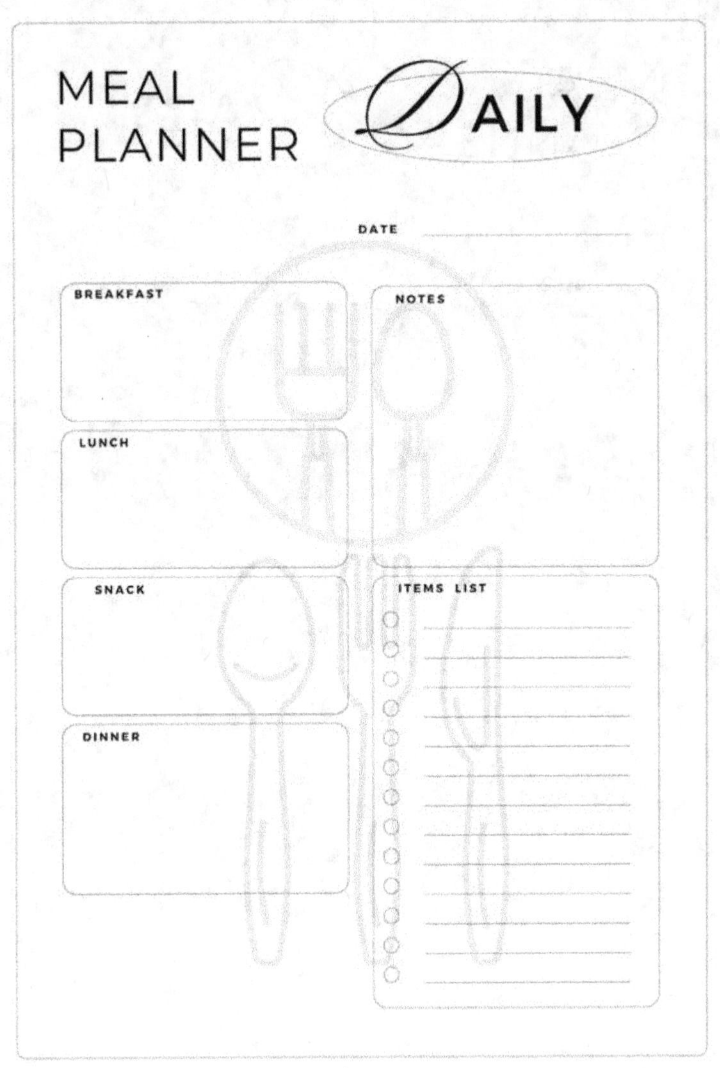

DAILY

DATE

BREAKFAST

NOTES

LUNCH

SNACK

ITEMS LIST

DINNER

MEAL PLANNER

DAILY

DATE

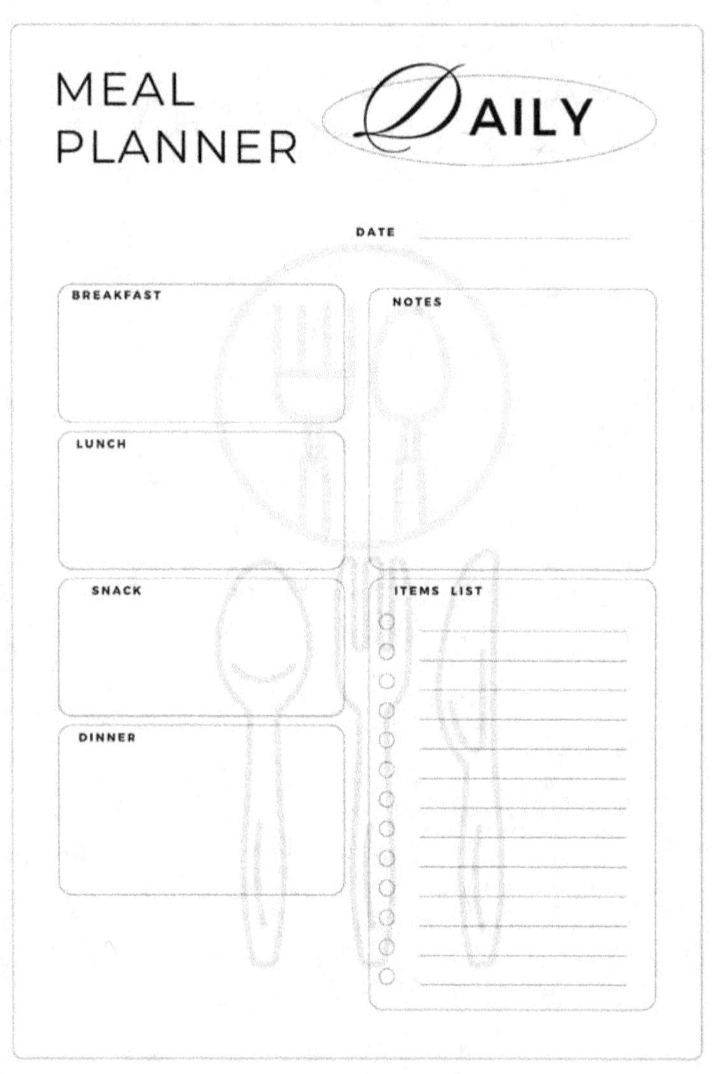

BREAKFAST

NOTES

LUNCH

SNACK

ITEMS LIST

DINNER

MEAL PLANNER

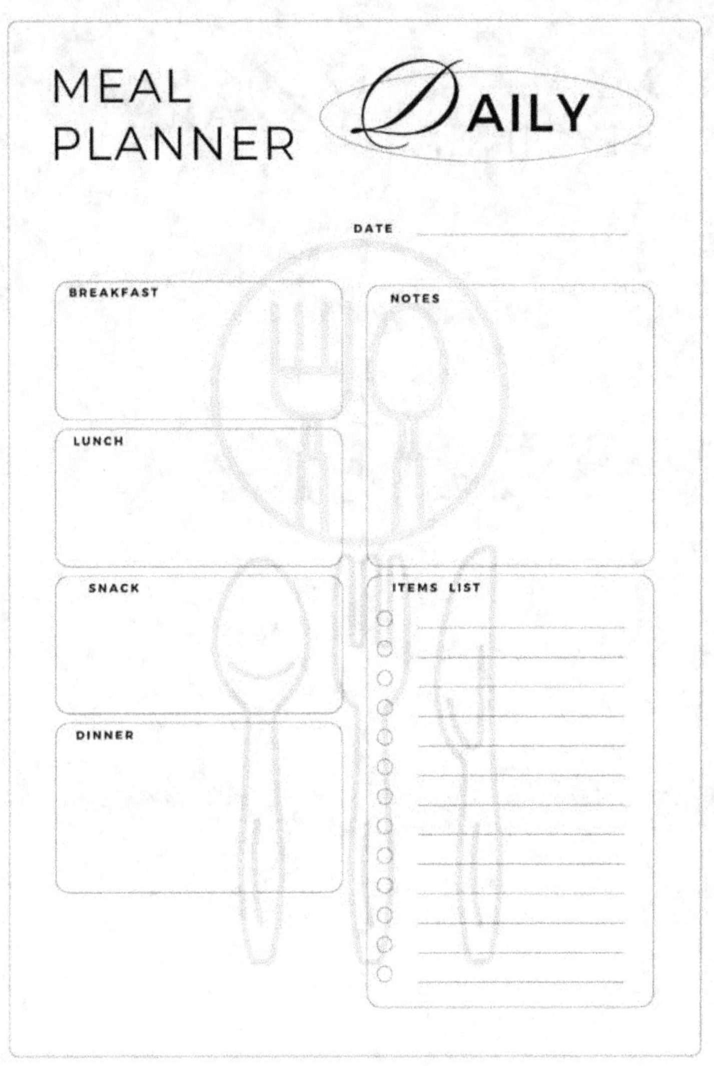

DATE

BREAKFAST

NOTES

LUNCH

SNACK

ITEMS LIST

DINNER

MEAL PLANNER

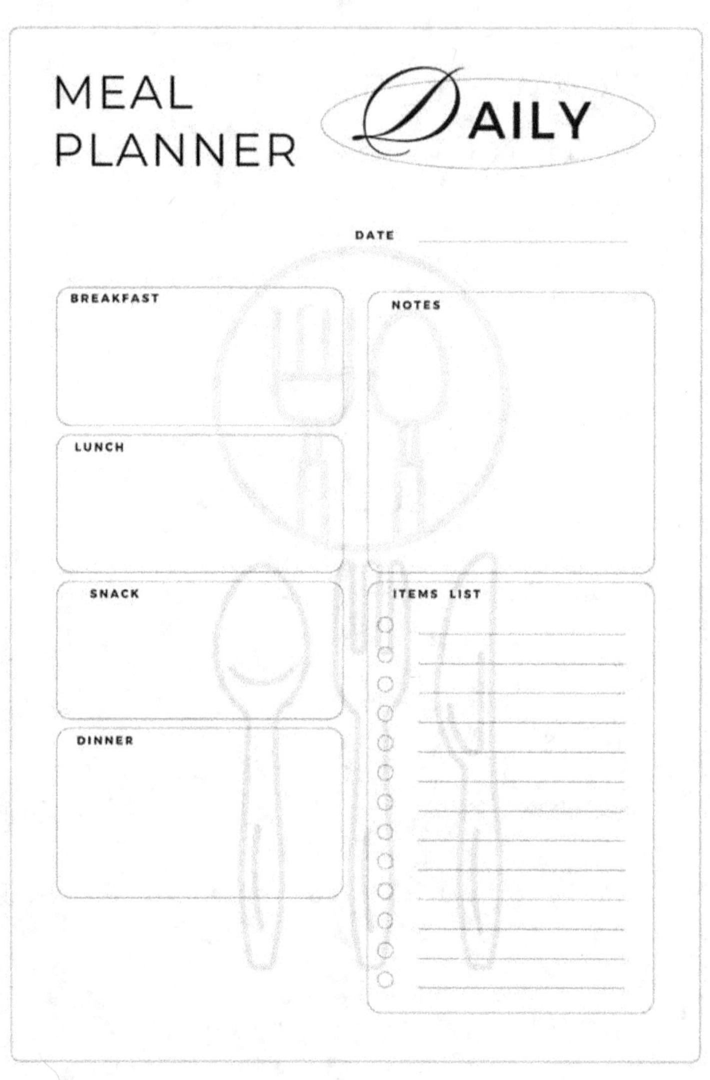

DAILY

DATE ______________________

BREAKFAST

LUNCH

SNACK

DINNER

NOTES

ITEMS LIST

MEAL PLANNER

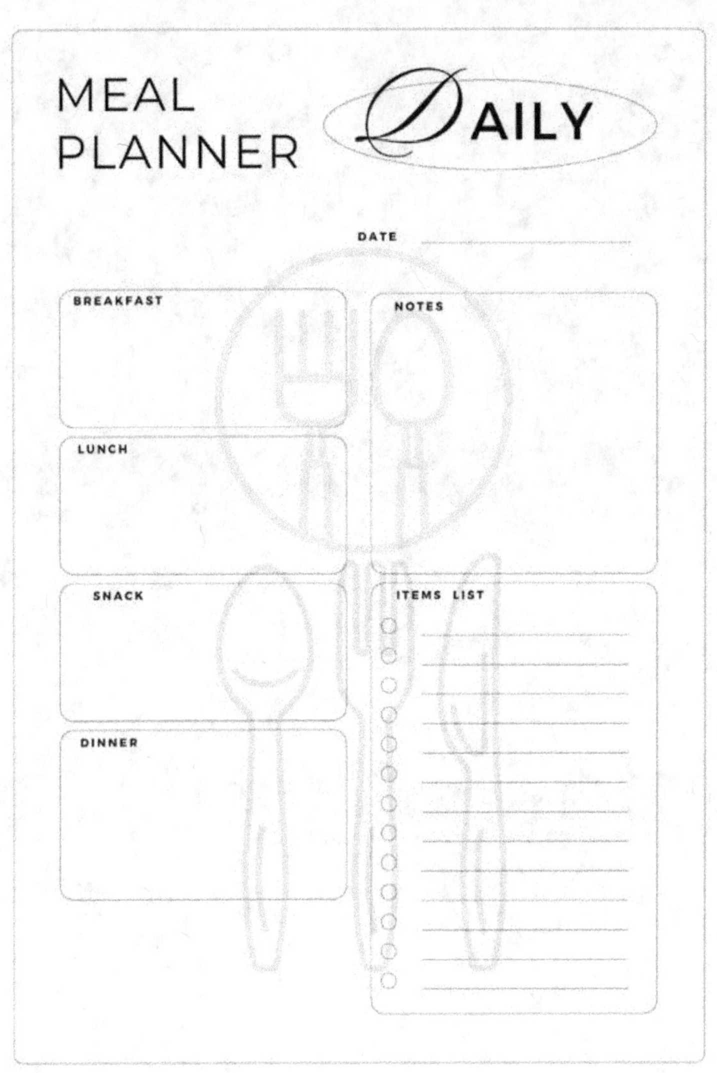